Sebastien,
Your Son

Claire Deveze

Sebastien, Your Son

Translated from the French
by Nathalie Arnaud

GREEN INTEGER
KØBENHAVN & LOS ANGELES
2006

GREEN INTEGER BOOKS
Edited by Per Bregne
København / Los Angeles

Distributed in the United States
by Consortium Book Sales and Distribution
1045 Westgate Drive, Suite 90,
Saint Paul, Minnesota 55114-1065
Distributed in England and throughout Europe by
Turnaround Publisher Services
Unit 3, Olympia Trading Estate
Coburg Road, Wood Green, London N22 6TZ
44 (0)20 88293009

(323) 857-1115 / http://www.greeninteger.com

First Green Integer Edition 2006
Published originally in French as
L'Encre de ta Mémoire: En hommage à Sébastien, ton fils
(Paris: L'Harmattan, 2002)
Copyright ©2002 by L'Harmattan
Published through arrangement with L'Harmattan
English language translation ©2006 by Nathalie Arnaud
Back cover copy ©2006 by Green Integer

The author would like to thank Vernon Henderson and
Marlene Willauer for their help in bringing this book to life,
and the always beloved support of Esther Kabbaz (in memoriam).

Design: Per Bregne
Typography & Design: Trudy Fisher
Cover Photograph: Claire Deveze

LIBRARY OF CONGRESS CATALOGING IN PUBLICATION DATA
Claire Deveze [1961]
Sebastien, Your Son
ISBN: 1-933382-08-2
p. cm — Green Integer 141
I. Title II. Series III. Translator

Green Integer books are published for Douglas Messerli
Printed in the United States on acid-free paper

Sebastien,
Your Son

— *It's not a story.*
  It's the tale of a sick child who dies.

— *So, it's a horrible story, even sadder than all*
  the others because it's a child who dies?

— *No, it's a story that inspires life. To give back*
  words to those who have lost them because
  they thought they were alone, because they
  thought that what they had lived was un
  speakable.

To Sebastien.
To Nathalie. To Guillaume and Pierre Alexis.

"It's only in absence that you can see well,
it's only when you miss someone
that you can express it well."
Christian Bobin

He is gorgeous; he's a beautiful child, fiery black eyes, and 10 years old. He's like that in the picture, the last picture of him, in his body, alive. The picture I love, it's at The Louvre, in February, it's cold, his cheeks are red, he holds my son Pierre by the shoulder, 10 years old, soon to be eleven.

He's gorgeous; he's a beautiful child, black eyes, fiery. They remained the same, up to the end, even when he was skinny, but still the same, Sebastien, smiling, when you don't recognize anything, but the flame in his eyes that says "Don't worry, I'm still here" and "Don't worry, I'm going to go, it hurts too much." And then he goes, just like he said he would in the interview with this student who came to see him in the hospital, three days before his death, at the Trousseau Hospital that Sunday in March, "You see, you shouldn't be afraid of sickness."

Your voice on the phone. It is filled with the light of Sebastien's eyes, with the heat of his skin. It doesn't cry; sadness gives it an amazing softness, a certain slow quality, too, when it says, "It's finished."

Sebastien dies the 11th of March 2001, at the Trousseau Hospital. He wanted the people he loved to be with him and he dies holding the hand of his father and his mother, who are reunited on that day.

He chooses a spring morning, the light toward which he used to turn more and more, the silence that he perceives beyond his hospital bed, and he dies bathed in the love of the people who love him, bathed in the infinite love of the life he's giving up slowly on this March morning.

I wasn't there.

It is your motherly words that, now and then, caress the surface; a few words pronounced randomly that I remember. I didn't even realize that I was memorizing them and they talk about the light he kept turning towards instead of looking at you, as if he were apologizing for not staying alive longer or as if he were regretting to leave you there, alive, with this impossibility to follow him and that suffering that you will inevitably suffer when he passes away. It is about that suffering that he is thinking, not his own: he wasn't thinking much about himself, and he was already gone under the effect of the morphine, but it is your suffering that he can't prevent. So he asks you to close the blinds, he looks at the window, turning away from your motherly stare, from this love that, more than anything else, prevents him from leaving, and he turns away his face so that you won't see the flame in his eyes die.

To give you the strength to go beyond his death, to live with his love, with his light, for life, yours.

You say, "It's over." I live in the United States, where it is Sunday morning, but for you it's the evening, and he died in France that afternoon. It's has been a long time that we have been friends, that I have seen the world through your eyes, your words; between us exists a bridge that was crossed long ago. I'm the one who called, you didn't try to reach me, you stayed motionless, frozen, completely focused on trying to keep living, to have arms that move, legs that walk, to breathe, just a little bit, a superficial breathing, that doesn't reach the depth of your despair. You have just lost everything at the same time: your sight, your words, your face, the right and the left side, your upper and your lower body parts. Complete internal bleeding: you have just lost a whole body, the body of your child and you're still alive. Doctors can't do anything for you. That's all you know in the state of complete anesthesia you're in.

I hang up the phone, in tears, while Pierre runs into my arms and says your name as if it were a question repeating several times: "Oh, no mom!" I hold him tight and we stay this way. It's our turn to be hit by this infinite sorrow, sorry that it is such a vast sadness, desperate to find out that it is even deeper each time we try to get relief. And this lasts

a long time, a time that has lost any reason to continue, in each other's arms, so close to the phone,
to you, to Sebastien. Your son, mine.

The following day, I come to join you, I am on a
plane, and I fly over Antarctica. *A beautiful trip* according to a magazine that I had read to Sebastien
in the hospital. I had told him about the ice, the
icebergs floating on the ocean and how beautiful
it was viewed from a plane, a glacier.

I cry in the darkness of the plane.

I arrive.

At the bottom of your building, there's a café. I greet the young woman who is washing glasses because you have told me about her great humor, about the words of encouragement she would throw at Sebastien when she saw him. She doesn't know me and answers me, a little bit surprised, with a little hand wave.

I don't walk up the six floors. I wait for the elevator that you had installed with the help of your father, because of all these renters' meetings and the estimate in the narrow cage of sickness, in the infinite smile of Seb, without windows or doors, on the heights of his laugh when he saw the elevator finished with such extraordinary delays. And it's a marvel that laugh, that I still hear in the stairway when he ran down the stairs with Pierre. They would calculate the number of stairs they could jump, with the sound of their shoes that would hit the wooden floors, all the way to the floors where you could hear their voices, talking too loudly, with a quick thought for some child who might be sleeping "Shush, there's a baby sleeping," and then again, on the second floor, they would burst out laughing: "The last one to get there is a loser!!"

I enter the elevator: I open the glass door; I smile,

as if Sebastien were welcoming me in his home. It's a funny cabin, tiny, built thanks to insane calculation, for a child that doesn't need it anymore. A great joke. A miraculous elevator that doesn't only go up the floors, but also elevates the heart, a machine, whose only purpose is to remind us of the one who needed it.

At the glass door, I suddenly hesitate to push the button, just like you hesitate to open a love letter written to someone who is not here anymore.

On the first floor is the building manager. She always had something sweet to say, one of these affectionate words that adults use sometimes and that children, because they hear it for the first time, literally grab.

The elevator goes up. On the third floor lives the old woman who congratulated him for being so tall when he helped her with her groceries, for being so strong, stronger than the front door that he would hold for her when she came back from the market, for being so courageous, when finally he would go up the stairs holding on to the rails like a mountaineer holds on to his rope. On the fifth floor, I remember Laurent, my husband, running to meet him, carrying him in his arms, him and his backpack, so light. I imagine you, carrying him on your back as if it were a game, the game of hide and seek on his mom's back. His little-prince face, half amused, half upset, just like this amazed look he loved so much. I see you carrying him more and more often, lower and lower, falling down the stairs, just like falling in love, agreeing to everything up to the last floor.

It's only recently that I have understood the battle for the stairs, this tough battle that the two of you had to fight for six months, in the trenches that were these stairs.

As the months went by, his body got lighter, his sickness got heavier like a stone on your shoulders. As the months went by, the battle between his love for you and his weakness, between his desire to protect you and the desire to be delivered, the same look, his face turned towards your face, talking, negotiating the stops: "OK, Mom, you carry me a little bit more and on the third floor, we stop."

You never told me about it.

But it probably wasn't easy with the tube in his chest, his chest that you had to be careful not to press, the effort you had to make to go up each step, making him believe that it wasn't that steep anymore. Sometimes you managed not to be out of breath, you calculated well how much energy you needed, so he would let you go on, shouting at you: "You're cheating!" to encourage you; sometimes you were having too much of a hard time so he would manage to go up a floor, in the middle of the climb, just giving you the time to catch your breath, and then vanquished, he would lie down again on your back, as if he were in a prairie on the side of a mountain, his head abandoned on the side of your shoulder. He was silent, his legs were dangling, as if they were already parting from his body, he would not protest anymore to hear you and you would climb to the top of the building. Some other times, you would carry him in front, as you did when he was three years old, five years old and he refused to walk, wanted to be carried, pretended to still be little, would ask for your arms, wanted you like you love when you're a child, when he would be away from you, on vacations with his grandparents at the ocean, at Tharon, and you would hold him firmly so you could still carry him, don't let your hands slip and tell him, one more time, the strength of your love for him, the child.

The elevator stops.
Sixth floor, you are here.
I would like to tell you beautiful things, but I don't know which ones. You're wearing a gray angora

sweater that looks very soft. I keep you in my arms, and we say nothing because no word can translate that feeling, our friendship, what I would like to be for you in these moments, your motherly love and suffering, this child taken away by death and who still says yes. And all these words that we don't say, all these words that I try to write today, that are dancing around, that surround us and prevent us from talking.

We sleep in the same bed.

It's not a bed; it's a room, mattresses arranged side by side. We all sleep in the bed he departed from, close to each other.

Everybody, they're all women. And this lasts a week.

A whole week during which we give each other infinite love, a love without measure. The kind of love reserved usually for children: a love above all else in the world. A love beyond the barriers of the body, that welcomes suffering even when it doesn't have the strength to ask for help, when it's hiding, when it isolates itself, fearing not to be understood. An infinite love, that doesn't count the hours, the days or the nights, available each second, awake, a love that has all the time, that doesn't ask for anything, that doesn't obey any desire, but the one that tries to stop sadness and solitude.

The first night you don't sleep, I have the feeling that in the darkness of the night you come into my arms each time I move, at each wave of sadness, going into Veronique's and coming back into mine. You put your face in the crook of my shoulder. You don't cry, I hear the perpetual movement of your tears inside you.

"If you love me, don't cry," you are the one who has chosen this opening statement for the church service.

To be there all the way, to be by your side, to cross over, even if we don't have a small boat, like in Egypt, to the side of the dead.

We are in the chapel of the hospital, like in the crypt of a tomb from the New Kingdom.

The child is lying down, his hands on his chest. His face has the softness of the painting on the walls of the tomb of that prince in the Valley of the Queens. His head shaved, symbol of royalty, he is covered in white and wears around his neck a mother of pearl necklace. A ray of sunshine. A reminder of his naked body, in the summer time. Like Carter discovering Tutankhamon's mummy and suddenly stopping his gesture when he revealed the neck of the young king, I contemplate the child and his necklace of white shells. A fabulous treasure, tons of pure gold, a sarcophagus that you have to open with ropes and suddenly a small crown of cut flowers made out of Egyptian papyrus and laid on the young prince's neck by a loving hand. A heavy wooden coffin, smothered cries, the gravity of a cold room, that is unfamiliar, and suddenly this necklace, a summer monsoon picked on the beach, a gift from his brother, Guillaume, that he would hold tight in his fists when he was asked to take it off in the hospital acknowledging the protection of his big brother and the magical virtues of this precious jewel that could heal.

Flowers, necklace, mother of pearl necklace, fragile, like a ray of sunshine, life around the neck, light. "If you love me, don't cry," it's difficult, but I'm willing to try to be as courageous as you, go to church, listen to the songs of the living, blessing the children in the crypt who draw hearts of all colors, thank his classmates who came to honor him with the light on their faces, so gentle, so calm, so eager to lay next to him the offering of a candle.

"If you love me, don't cry" forgive him, it's the priest who cries in the cemetery, it's so beautiful to see a priest who cries to communicate with his heart and his thoughts, facing the open tomb, tears that he doesn't try to hide, tears which we don't know whether they are shed for the child's body given to the earth or for the love expressed in words that day.

The day in your apartment, a lot of people around you, your older son, children, friends, your family, a lot of silence, relevant words coming from the bottom of hearts.

We go out, go for a walk in a park to clear your bleary eyes. It's true that it's springtime. A man walking by stops and offers to take our picture in front of a tree. He didn't see our sadness, only our transparency, our true presence in the alleys with this attention we have for the daylight, the noise of the leaves in the wind, the flowers. This awareness that we were alive, that we were walking, existing.

The same night returns.

You fall asleep. Maybe it is the medications.

Ariane, your first friend who pops in my memory, turns toward me. She's more than a friend, an associate, your ally in this amazing project that you started in Paris: a silent universe, but busy with desks where I would sneak in sometimes to steal a lunch with you. She doesn't say anything, puts her hand on my shoulder and takes me in her arms.

I open the book of tears to any page haunted by images of Sebastien present, coming through the door, asking me: "Why don't grown ups play in the woods, why do they simply walk, are they not allowed?" They 're not words, they're laughs, the tree where he was seated to talk to me about the happiness in his life, about the clear sound of mint tea that they pour in Morocco, by dropping it from high above into golden glasses, about the Sahara dunes, with the sand that crumbles under one's feet, but if you walk fast, you get there, you can get to the top of the dune, ". . . not everyone you know, but I could," it's a huge wave of sadness and at the same time a happy thought for you, Seb.

It's difficult, but we can do it, something in you insists, something that pushes me, to write this book like a gift that you would have left me. I still hear Laurent pouring the tea into those golden glasses on the 31st of December 1999, when it was not yet the year 2000, I still see the expression of your happy face, your compliments to Laurent for this magical table, it's true that you loved beautiful tables. "Party" you said, so Laurent added little glass candle holders with petite snow stars that drew on the tablecloth silver reflections, embroidered napkins, dead leaves picked up in the woods, pine cones, all enveloped in Christmas decorations. He told you the story of the blue crystal glasses brought back from Poland; your eyes wide while he pretended that they gave a better taste to the water.

It was the first time that we celebrated New Year's

Eve with the family, parents and children reunited, instead of the usual party reserved for the adults when we would dance and go to bed in the morning. With the family, it only meant us. I can't help thinking it was a premonition. First, the storm and that epic return trip across France without electricity, restaurants closed on the highway, the plastic of greenhouses torn, the trees broken, signs thrown on the street, night everywhere, Paris lost far away, inaccessible, and finally the house, just in time to celebrate with you this first of January 2000 that we had talked about for years and that seemed like an impossible date to attain in the present, but forever in the future. And here we were, all of us together. Laurent was setting up the table, was folding the napkins in the glasses while we were waiting for you and the two boys. I rode to town to get coquilles St. Jacques forgetting that the two boxes would not fit in the basket. You arrived while I was gone; I rang the bell accompanied by two men I met on the road who gave me a ride home. We laughed, the children had put on bow ties to please us, and white shirts over their jeans, Pierre was putting too much cream on his salmon slices, Sebastien was scolding him because he would spill some and wasn't eating properly, far away we heard the fireworks that were kissing the Eiffel Tower, we didn't go out, we danced, drank cider in cups that looked like jewels.

Ariane goes through the thickness of my silence and settles in the middle to give me her eyes as a mirror.

Five days.

It's today's date. We are five days after Sebastien. Friday.

Days don't count anymore. From now on, we should count in centuries that separate the past from the future, in abysses that separate the before from the after. Or should it be in toys, in clothes, in books that remind us of him. So few things, so light, so easy to fold, and put away.

In the evening, after school, his friends come, little boys and little girls who are ten years old. They go into the bedroom as if they were just visiting him, looking for encouragement when they go in, looking around them to understand his absence.

Your elder son signals to them to choose an object. "You will do this in memory of me," they are Christ's words, and they are the priest's words during mass. Your son doesn't say anything, takes on to the end his big brother role, tries not to forget anybody during the offering, accompanies them to the door. At the end, he takes into the closet a piece of clothing, a few toys, puts his hand in mine, leans against my shoulder, asks me to take away what's left — when I can, when I have time — gives me a kiss before joining his dad for the weekend.

You too, you come into the room. You too, are here, obligated to look at the end of the world, forced to choose what you want to keep from the past, from your sacrificed child with this wound that prevents you from breathing. In your eyes is the pain of extreme love. You would like to lay down here, on the bedroom carpet, not to move anymore, relieve this pain in the heart of your belly that rips you apart, scream, shout maybe, but no. You stay still, standing, your life requires that you stay standing, that you persevere, that you still carry your eldest, your family, your mother, that you continue to exist to show them that you can still walk, that a present is possible.

For the first time and without really thinking about it, it is to Sebastien that you turn, you ask him for help. You call on his generosity, the plastic dinosaur that he gave a child he didn't know, the reassuring gestures that he made to his neighbors in the hospital, his willingness to be the first one on the phone to say "How are you?" to the attention he was giving others when he realized that sickness was making people aggressive, capricious, that sickness multiplied sadness with being tired. You remember his first weeks of treatment, his first sufferings, his first desires impossible to fulfill, his first tantrums, his first words he used to talk about his body, to manifest and to share the pain, and then his efforts to protect his loved ones, to shut up the sadness. The way he said he was less sick than others, "I'm lucky, I just have leukemia," this way he talked, this way he jumped above the pain, trying to go over it. You see him bringing his collection of soccer magazines to the hospital, putting aside the chocolate cream from his lunch for his brother: "Guigui, I have goodies for you." Gifts too. A wallet and a key chain with a silver bear on it, bought for the thirteenth birthday of Guillaume, at the end of March.

You break the silence, you show me the room and you tell me to give everything away.

I ask to make sure I understand. "Everything?" And you tell me "Yes, everything. To children."

I don't know if Sebastien is giving you a sign, congratulating you in silence, telling you that it's good, that it is the way to heal.

It seems to me that you could stay there for hours looking at him, close the door, stay alone with him in this room.

Forbidding entrance to anybody.

You do the opposite. I understand the cost of your footsteps to get out of the room like you would turn your back on someone you love.

After a few minutes, without a warning, without a sound, you collapse.

It's as if you were suddenly stuck by an invisible sword and you just understood the void, the separation a second time. Or as if, once and for all, you let the pain go through you, a pain that you can no longer hold back and to which you surrender completely.

And the pain comes with the violence of a barbaric horde that hid for a long time, it steps all over your will, sets on fire everything from your stomach to your lips, burns your insides, pierces the surface of your skin. You shout, you fall down, emptied of all your substance, your body shaken with spasms as if you were about to die at our feet, disappear, laying on a wound that is ripping you apart, your head on the pillow, taken by despair.

Nothing can stop this sudden drop: not Veronique's arms that embrace you, not my caresses on your hair, not the reassuring words that Ariane whispers to you. It's your body that, this time, despairs, and we stay at the surface, weak, taking turns to relieve your pain.

Veronique gets up and I take her place: I lay down by your side, I hold up your head, I hold you in my arms and I hold you against my heart. I close my eyes, I feel the wave of tears shake my shoulder, I welcome your pain, my hand holds your arms a little bit tighter to prevent it from taking you away, and I let it go, I don't do anything to stop it from overwhelming you, I leave your face drowned in the silence of the room, I kiss you, I hold your legs with my own to prevent the shaking of your whole body, I cry so that my cries put a stop to yours, I whisper in your ear sweet words that you don't hear; I tell you about the Mediterranean sky with the pink and blue shades, the gray Parisian sky, the sun on the Pacific Coast, The Little Prince of Saint-Exupéry and his stars' migration, and you fall into the darkness, lonely, far, while, without any power, I wait on the side giving you my hand.

Ariane comes into the room, she kneels at the foot of the bed, takes care of your lower body, lays on your legs and massages them, in silence, while I continue, tirelessly, to rock you and hold you tight. Now and then, she looks up at me to share the beats of her heart, to harmonize it with mine, with yours, with the blood that runs through the veins in the time of that room. Then Veronique comes back, takes your head back in her arms, or it's me, or it's Ariane. Sometimes, one of us gets up, prepares the meal, sets the table, another takes her place, kisses a strand of your hair, draws signals that will bring you back to life.

Slowly you can walk, go all the way to the table,

open your eyes slowly as if you had to adjust to the daylight, after a long night. On the plate, something to eat. You don't touch anything. We play love songs, a really old record that talks about the eternity of life, about passion, about death. Veronique and I know the words, we sing old tunes to make the meal lighter, like a shower of minuscule piano keys on your face to wash away the despair.

Ariane listens to us, wrapped in the silence of a smile that seems like a response to the words of the song.
She puts the fork in your hand, you learn again the gesture you have to make to use a fork, to bring the food to your lips.
You eat love songs with a little bit of food.

Saturday.

It's my turn to obey, I go to the edge of the world, and I go into the little one's bedroom. A word that's written everywhere, on the walls that you had re-decorated a few months earlier to make it a "grown up room," on the bed sheets, the stuffed animals, in the library where are stacked all the stories read and all the books that were offered to him. I open one; it's a book of photography. Inside a few words of your aunt Maya who talks to him about travels and exoticism. I open another one, I picture you bending over him, sitting on the side of his bed, with your voice when he looked at your face, happy to feel you so close.

I open the window, I sit on the bed and I stay there, in the time of death not yet unraveled. The weather is nice; I realize that I'm looking at the clouds run-ning in the sky leaving some spots of blue shade. It seems to me that you are somewhere in this in-finity of blue. "In Normandy at the seaside" Veronique, who took you there, told me, away from this room where I'm going to organize objects that could kill you in the light of your present absence. On the wall, facing me, there are pictures taken in the desert in Morocco, a dune, the fine sand and Sebastien as a Touareg. On a shelf, a collection of iron soccer players that the nanny who took care of him as a child, will come later to get with open hands, shaking, as if the pain had suddenly made her blind.

I don't dare touch anything, I go out, I walk on the sidewalks of Avenue des Ternes, I don't go into the stores since he didn't have permission to go in: "My days are free, but what do you want to do all alone walking in the streets?" I picture the room inch by inch, the miniature white limousine, one of our last gifts to make him dream, set on the desk, the poster of Tintin, the school bag, the school agenda desperately blank, the pencil case that Pierre asked to inherit. Empty catalog and yet each object opens an abyss.

The cell phone in my pocket rings, the worried voice of Ariane, she reminds me of the time, the meeting set in the apartment to help me move. She doesn't hang up right away, asks me to look around me, to find the name of the street, and tells me how to get back.

I come back.

This time, I pass the bed, I go all the way to the big white closet that you bought to make the room cleaner, "Not a germ" you said laughing, you made fun of me, of you, of our past disorders, of the dust that we didn't see and that we were now chasing around. I open the closet; you didn't have time to fix the drawer's handles.

I start to put things in order, I put the knights back in their castle, the castle back in the box bought a few days before his death, when you knew he was lost, when you would have bought him all the knights on earth, to give him more moments of life, of happiness. I carry the magical box in my arms: "he came out of his bed" you told me, "he got up to open his gift." I lay the box on the floor as delicately as possible, I put the knights with the others, all the others, the space warriors, those from Star Wars and those from the cartoons, the Batman, the changing robots, men, animals, the "heroes" he called them. I recognize the soldiers, the cops, the tanks, the ambulances, the jeeps, and the motorcycles. I think about the message he left you on your answering machine the day you offered them to him, a song with invented words, a melody for you both with his voice, just a gift, for nothing, just for you mom, free, just to thank you, sleep well, you see I sing, I'm happy, toys are enough to erase the sickness. "I would like you to see my army" he wrote to Pierre. I stop, I picture them facing each other in the bathtub with toy in each hand, here a plane, there a hero, both telling each other the same story, conquering an invisible citadel, under-standing each other just with sounds and hand gestures, to signal the beginning of the battle, in-terrupt by big splashes of water. Usually the noise would grab my attention: after several unsuccess-ful final assaults, I ended up showing up asking for peace talks to avoid flooding. They kept apolo-gizing and begging me to give them a few more minutes, promising to be quiet.

I suddenly think about your bathroom, about the heroes maybe abandoned upstairs. I run, I rush up the stairs before forgetting, I find three on the side of the bathtub, I stop, I tip my head, I lean against the door and I hold in my hands the three little colorful men, symbols of a recent past that I hold a few more seconds. I cry. I think about this Bradbury novel where firemen start fires. I don't put things away, I erase. With the walks in the Fontainebleau forest when he would jump from rock to rock, with the soccer matches our sons played together, with the roller blade parties where he would complain about the roads, I organize a box of "outside toys," with the afternoons of sickness spent on the floor on his room's carpet building towns and villages, I make a box of "inside toys."

Then the clothes, the dance of gifts, the outings, the holiday memories, the birthdays and the Christmas past. It's the more difficult, so I don't look, I pack in the emergency of a calendar that destroys itself.

Others joined me: your family, and always Ariane who kneels next to me to help me. A whole army that organized itself with precise gestures, short sentences, to mask the hesitations of the voice and the hands, your niece with the tape, the markers always lost, your sister who is thinking about such and such toy for such and such child in such and such orphanage, the brother and the brother-in-law who combine their pain to move the toy closet into the hall. At the end, there's nothing left. The boxes took everything away. The room seems suddenly seized by the gravity of the silence. Your sister says that she won't give everything away right away, that she will wait a little longer. We put in the room other objects and other pieces of furniture to keep it from being empty.

I set aside for you a little box with his favorite toys, a little penguin, turtle and plastic warriors, some softness and strength.

Suddenly I feel the weight of the trip, the jetlag and the breadth of the distance crossed.

I go back to America.

If you love me don't cry, I obey, I write.

For you. Mother, woman, lover, little girl, friend, love, words are not catching up to you whose smile I only remember, the eyes, the smile in the eyes and your look that moves me.

For you. And I write it. It's difficult to be as big as you. As big as love. Not to wait for anything so that everything is light. To abandon yourself to the world, to the agile innocence of the water, to the Santa Ana and to the wind of the sea, the one that dries laundry and brings the rain. To look at life passing through, in the world's nets.

My son Pierre often picks up rocks, anywhere, it must be because of his name all those stones that I find everywhere in the house, in his desk's drawers, in his school bag, in the pockets that I empty before I put his laundry in the machine. It's amazing all those stones that he collects. His favorites are smooth, round, those river stones, chosen in the middle of the waters as if they were diamonds, and that he brings back so proudly in his hands, always a little bit disappointed when they dry. But he also likes the lava rocks, the brown ones, the "naked ones," the "not pretty ones," those that have a strange shape, those that don't, the "normal ones" like he says, and ultimate happiness, a shell fossil discovered a summer day on a grapevine wall. Sebastien liked stones, I didn't know it. I knew he was a collector. He loved even the word "collection" and used it for everything: one precious object, a unique picture and it was a world of happiness, of joy, a collection.

With Pierre they collected subway tickets. They had every kind, some almost new picked up in trash cans in subway stations, some really dirty, picked up on the sidewalk even though there was dust, the shoes' marks or the grease, all used, of all colors, even if the subway cards were their favorite. They refused to throw them away even when I said something, even when I threatened, finding them lying down on the bed with clean sheets looking at the dates and the destinations, thrown by so many people, the fingers stained by the ink of the validation machines. And one should have seen the pride with which Seb would give Pierre, who had just moved to Paris, handfuls of these confetti of a new kind, the use of which was obvious to both of them. And that's why it was fascinating to me to see these two children, one Parisian, the other not, willing to gather these tickets that nobody else wanted.

They didn't organize them by date or destinations, they were satisfied making piles of them and counting them. In Paris, you told me about this stone in a heart shape that you gave to Seb, you opened your wallet to show it to me, it was a lava rock, smooth. You showed it to me like others show their child's most recent picture.

You lost it, you just wrote that to me. The wallet when you were shopping, the stone, the whole collection all at once. You collect his love, free from all reality, light.

They said about each other:
"My friend for life."

Pierre doesn't tidy up his room; he is not a clean child, not a clean freak. You gave him a few of Seb's toys, he takes care of them. He says: "If he comes back, he'll be able to find everything."

His friend for death too.

He keeps on loving him, he keeps on talking to him with words forbidden by grown ups:

"Hang in there pal, I'm here."

As if this could protect him, protect both of them from this terrible thing that makes adults cry and spare them. I sit on the bed, and I talk to him gently:

"You know that he's not coming back?"
He shrugs and doesn't answer me, he knows it, but beyond this knowledge he can still hear his friend answering him, he keeps playing on his bed with little plastic people, and as much as I want to be the mother and the grown up, they are both playing, laughing, imagining battle plans, talking and closing the door to have peace.

Sebastien was a little bit bigger than Pierre, it shows in the pictures, he was six months older, it's true. Like him, he was thin, smooth skin, with long and lean muscles, well defined. They liked to play soccer, wear champion's jerseys, take off their shirts, side by side, and compare their chests. They loved lying down on couches, on the floor, when the parties would go on, and they wanted to let us know that it was late, that they were tired.
They were not good students, serious, conscientious, no competition between them, and no school gossip.
One time only, they recited to each other poems learned in school, going over them, happy to see that they still knew them and laughing about the fact that they recited them out loud. It's a Sunday, it's the first time that Sebastien sleeps over since we have come back to Paris, we are in a train that

runs between Paris and Versailles and Pierre is amazed at the new RER train with decks. Sebastien is thrilled, he pulls on the sleeve of my coat, and we all go up to the second deck, we find four seats available next to the window on the right. We look outside the window looking at the houses that pass by, Paris and this incredible luck to be together. Sebastien is sitting next to me, he has beautiful brown eyes, long eyelashes, I look at him the way you look at people you love, detailing, amazed at the slightest detail of his physique, his hands are still small, but the fingers are long and thin, the softness of the skin on his cheeks still full above his smiles, his round ears, rounder than Pierre's, I tell them, I put their heads closer, one blond the other dark haired, they laugh, they catch each other's ears, examine their ear lobes, joke "you see, we're the same."

I call him my little Bastien, he talks, he has a thousand things to tell me, to explain to me, about his life that "is not so easy," and he says everything with such simplicity, with sentences that start with "you see" asking Pierre to be his witness. He puffs his chest out, he's wearing a black and yellow jacket that you just bought him, I remember because you gave me the address so I could buy the same for Pierre, because the winter here is cold, I mainly remember because I picture him reciting out loud a poem about the moon, a Sunday, on a train, in Paris, the three of us.

Pierre doesn't pay attention; he doesn't listen to what we tell him. Since Sebastien has been sick, he has become completely deaf to the world. I had to go to the school: his teacher was worried about what he referred to as "his absences." He thought that it could be a condition that hadn't been diagnosed, advised me to have his ears tested, and because the tests didn't reveal anything, the eyes "children that are distracted are sometimes nearsighted" he told me.

Pierre doesn't have any problems with his eyes. He is sad, that's all, and to the question "why?" he answers "all the time." His sadness is timid, silent, and almost invisible. It's also tragic like this Christmas even when he played with other children and missed, not on purpose, the slide on which he climbed.

He doesn't say that he's hurting, not even during the needle shots, at the hospital, or at wake up time when he refuses the gifts that the nurse is bringing him. He explains to me that he's not really sick, not for real, asks me to give the gifts to the children who are going to be there for a long time, the children "who are prisoners there," the ones who are suffering. He is happy to be in bed, to eat mashed potatoes, to ask questions about the wires, the medical equipment, to play his video games with one hand: "You see? With only one hand, it's possible!" He ends up opening a gift, thanks to the nurse who is so nice. It's a little stuffed orange dog. We keep it preciously. It's a little bit Sebastien's.

In February, you send me pictures. Sebastien is having fun with the wires, the intravenous tubes, he sticks his tongue out, makes faces on his hospital bed, and he's playing.

They are pictures that deny the sickness. But it's there, everywhere.

Seb is washing himself with a friend, and the picture only shows his legs, so skinny that you have this thought that comes with tears, when you see that in spite of everything, he still is able to stand up. Seb smiles and you cry seeing him smile in spite of the dark circles, and this face marked by exhaustion.

It's looking at these pictures that makes Pierre suddenly wants to talk to him. For months he refuses, he can't, he can't bring himself to break the confidence that he has in Seb's strength, this silent promise they made each other not to worry, to despise the sickness, because they're ten years old and at ten years old you don't die, you're invincible, and also because, Pierre tells me, "it's the good guys who win against the dark forces in Star Wars, and Sebastien is a good guy, I know him."

He calls a first time.

The first time you wrote to me: "They might not know what to say to each other," but Seb recognizes his voice right away as if they were simply continuing a conversation started a few minutes earlier. They chat.

When they talked for the last time, it was about fishing I think. At the end, they said "bye" and hung up.

Sebastien, it's a pretty name. It makes you think about this TV show that went on and on, about this little boy who runs, with his dog, in the mountains, free, happy in this. That's how I picture him, running in the fields of Brittany with this brilliant smile that's so unique to children.

You write to me that the cops fined you yesterday because you hadn't passed the smog check. They don't know that mothers who run to hospitals don't have the time to take care of that kind of thing. I feel like writing to them, making a connection between these two worlds: the outside world, the alive one, quick, with work and summer, the taxes and the news, the wasted time and the other, the inside world, motionless, with its colored doors, its floors, its protocols, its intravenous tubes, its machines that ring night and day, its I.V. drip, precious. You don't have time to sleep, you don't have time to swallow the sandwiches that we sometimes bring you in the dining room reserved for the parents, for the mothers, mainly the mothers because fathers don't know that children can die, you don't have the heart to eat what he would love to eat and this week it's forbidden, "This week, he can't have pickles, ham, salmon or anything that's salty," you don't have the heart to lie to him, you don't have the heart to leave him before he falls asleep, you don't know how to have a heart anymore, a body, you can't sleep, fall asleep knowing that he's alone in his bed, you don't have time to go work, to take care of your house, to be alone, to be sick. You only have him in this world, you take him in your arms, you talk to him, you bathe him, you massage his legs, you're pregnant again, you carry him, you could carry him to the end of times. Do you remember when he was just born? You were calling me, you were laughing, "we should hurry up, he doesn't leave me alone," and we would hurry, and we talked about them, our babies, yours, and mine. And we would hurry to change their diapers, to feed them, to rock them to sleep, so that they wouldn't cry alone in their bed, so that their little behinds wouldn't get hurt, we would rub cream on them, we would rub their hair with almond oil, we would anoint, soap and perfume the little bodies, we would take the tiny little hands to put them in the pajamas without forgetting a finger, we would breast feed, we would contemplate the little round face resting in our hands, perfectly content. Your baby. Mine too, a little bit, sometimes I would keep him, I took care of his well being. Sebastien is sleeping, and it's the same child you tuck in bed, you kiss, you envelop in the threads and the sheets of his hospital bed. Your baby. You give him everything and he takes everything like the rest, with an infinite softness, he is giving himself.

He gives everything. At the beginning, a few days of his life per week, his hair, most of his toys that might contaminate him, water, since the water from baths is forbidden, the water from small showers and the one from the pools he dreamt about, his clothes that are now too big because of the list of foods that are forbidden. But it's not enough, the sickness wants more, it invents words, new rules, a new schedule: "public places, school, museums, subways are forbidden," it adjourns things, cancels the play dates, imposes new paper clothes, hospital clothes, it takes away his books, his school bag, his favorite meals, and at the end, it takes away his dreams and his little boy's desires: the soccer games with friends, the walks in the forest, his bike, the holidays at the seaside, the fishing trips, the postcard collections and the trips to the end of the earth "especially in the desert, I like deserts." Everything. The sickness wants everything. His arms, his leg, the entire right side. And what he doesn't know, an adult body, children, a man's future. And he gives it everything, without crying, lying on his bed, motionless, until there's nothing left but his love, the one thing that death has left him.

Suddenly, you have the time.

Time doesn't matter anymore. The cops stop you at the gates of the city, talk to you about the year that has just passed without you, without smog check. And we laugh about the joke of this life that goes on.

One after another, there are three of us taking turns next to you, looking after your heart emptied of its light. You are in pain; it's like you are on a dark path and we are walking by your side, warning you about the obstacles.

After I left, Veronique stayed another week, she's the fire that illuminates your presence now and then, for the duration of a weekend, of a few days, she takes you to Italy, feeds your desire to live. Ariane is there every day; she is the bread and the water you get your nourishment from. She stays at your place a few days, she doesn't know how long, she's not counting. The time necessary to help you go back to work, eat, sleep, go out in the street, shop. I write. You answer. I read your letter in the morning, I read it at night, late, when the children are asleep, when the tiredness settles in and I can't do anything else but read, let my fingers run on the keyboard.

I only write the breath of fresh air, the sun light when it's morning, the orange sky at sunrise: sweet words, tender words. "A real joy to read your words before I go to bed after having worked so many hours in front of my computer. A backache, my hands hurt, but you just healed everything. Tender kisses."

I try to create with my absent voice a space, a shelter, a cradle, a refuge to welcome your words. I'm far away, absent yet still present, like Sebastien probably is, I try to harmonize my voice to his.

I listen, I don't leave you, and I write to you morning and night, I write to you endlessly, I tell you to look towards the sky.

You often stumble. Sometimes, just a water puddle or a wet sidewalk is enough, and suddenly you picture Sebastien adjusting his cap under the rain with this eyebrow movement that either says that he's smiling or that he's about to ask a question, because his cap is too big, his scalp nude, passersby were about to turn around or the sun was cascading on his visor. Sometimes, it's a sad word from someone who doesn't know, who asks you if you have children, how many children you have and you don't answer, you don't know how to answer, you don't know how to deal with the absence. Sometimes it's the look in the eyes of a happy child, smiling, giving his hand in confidence, and who walks on the edge of your eyes, sometimes it's because of a tree, the woods, the forests, the squares where you took him, away from the city and the forbidden public places, sometimes it's because of the time and all this extra time, this time after, terribly slow, sometimes it's because of the days: the painful dates make the weather of probable storms and the storms come inevitably. And there's always an object, a song, a favorite color, the saltshaker on the table and he couldn't have salt.

It's an intelligent child, he knows how to send you messages and you smile because sometimes I hear them at the same time you do.

Summer comes.

With summer, my return and the house in France at the seaside.

Sebastien liked it, this house on the Mediterranean. This is the place I was telling him about last year, in July, this last summer when I didn't know it was the last, when I thought it was just about helping him overcome a few weeks, a few months maybe of being in the hospital: it's strange, I was never afraid for his body, I was afraid that his childhood might get damaged, his imagination, his confidence. I was wrong, he was never desperate.

A doctor told me recently that his death was predictable, he had seen all the first test results, "he had one in ten chances to heal." He was not talking to me, he was adamant, as if his numbers were reassuring him, helped him accept death, inevitable, since it was already present on paper right from the beginning of the sickness. I never thought about your death Sebastien, I only spent two weeks by your side, but I never doubted that you would heal, just like all the others who took turns at your bedside: those who kept giving you French and Math lessons for your future, those who knew how to tell fairy tales improvising each moment, changing the story depending on your mood, for your present of being a little boy, those who would watch

TV with you, so that you were not alone, those who would come talk to you and you're the one who listened to them, those who tried to bring you something to eat that you would like in spite of your diet that changed every day, something that would have put a stop to this terrible weight loss, not because you didn't want to eat, actually food had become an obsession, but they were trying to feed you and not the sickness, going through the supermarket aisles, with the list of forbidden foods in one hand and in the other the grocery bags, cooking at any time of the day or night.

You join me.
We have children, mine, yours, the living and the absent; a lot of meals to prepare, of food to choose from the markets, of clothes to wash, of laundry to iron, of walks, of showers, of words you have to be careful about, of goodnight kisses, of goodnight kisses to keep, for the child who is not here, who can't receive them. The infinity of the pain, the love. That starts over every day. Sometimes like a fatality that you don't want to flee, you are absent, absorbed by your pain, taken really far from yourself. I offer you the refuge of my arms as the storm is raging and is knocking you down, absorbs all your

energy, keeps you from getting any rest. I wait. I walk with you on the beach. I look for the path between the sand and the strength of the waves. I look at you and your eyes are far away like prisoners of images that I don't know, of far away lands. My words die on the beach, I lose them one by one. I welcome a pain emptied of all words.

You like Pierre a lot.
It's astonishing, this son whom I impose on you and who's not yours.
Sometimes I'm afraid that you will lose it, sometimes I would like to stop Pierre's eyebrows when he moves them, astonished, with this naïve air, childlike, disarming, the same that Sebastien had. Sometimes I look at him and I don't try to stop him from being ten years old, from asking questions, from being surprised, from laughing, and liking mother-of-pearl necklaces, even if it's the same that Sebastien was wearing during his last earthly trip.

"One of the two was saved," it's what is written in the Bible. One was saved and not the other. Which one of the two, my friend, which one of the two, and if it's yours, mine, why him?

I try to distract you from your pain. I try to make you think about futile things, take you away from him, the lost child, to help you close this gap inside you, rebuild yourself. I give you my hand, when we walk, at night, along the empty streets next to the villas. We walk far, like people who don't have a goal. I tell you stories. The one about the tree of words in Africa under which people talk to make sure they have said everything before they die, the one about the moon, so pretty in its little dress when it falls in the sea and see how round is the moon, so beautiful tonight as it bathes in the horizon.

You say it's difficult.

On the sand, you picture Sebastien at five years old, little warrior, sitting alone, looking at the other children of the beach club exercising and asking "why do we have to do this and that?" You don't say anything and we stay, wrecked in the middle of the beach, in the middle of the night, on the horizon a light is sending a message, red light, green light, and I don't know how to make you feel better.

You try your best to mask your sadness, but your eyes are tired and swollen. You cry on your bed when I close the door, when driving your car, in the water of the ocean and while doing the dishes, when you think you're alone, and when you're with me. You cry on rainy days, "because," you say laughing, "it's raining in my heart." You recite Verlaine to pretend, and you cry on sunny days because he loved the heat and the blue skies as Moustaki was singing on the radio "I love you as much as I loved you, but I can't say it now."

"All the tears in your body," that's how you say it, at home in the south of France. Familiar tears. It's mine, you're crying, tears for all the mothers, it's how my heart bleeds when I worry, when my children are sick, have a cold, when they have a stomachache, when they're worried, when they change school, when there's an airplane strike and that they call me from a hotel frightened.

It seems that you're smiling. Your face is serene, motionless, no traces of pain. You don't want people to be sad for you. Anybody. Not you, not anybody. Not me, not others. Those who don't know, who wouldn't know what to say, those who are not close, those who are shy, those who waited too long to talk to you and who won't do it anymore, the parents waiting outside the school, the merchants, the colleagues.

How can you tell them that his voice still resonates inside you when you hear "hospital," when I'm talking about a hotel?

How do you tell them to go beyond your face, to go towards you with simple words, clear words, that are not afraid to be clumsy, without an effort in the air and the silence, let the sun in by opening wide the doors, like right after a storm?

I write, I try to understand.

To measure the absence. "The three of us," you would say. The sadness of these four words, the pain of the number three from now on forbidden. Life suddenly overwhelming. The car with its seat ridiculously small, too narrow for Sebastien to sleep with the cover and the pillow prepared for him, the endless care you had for his body to rest, so that he falls asleep inside your thoughts, the way you worried about him on these long trips to the hospital or the sea, in Normandy where you managed to take him in spite of it. A back seat really too big, too large now, a real desert, a cold space you're trying to avoid, maybe to imagine it sometimes, asleep in the back. The house emptied of its meaning, the boys' floor that has become the boy's floor. The rooms' doors that we don't close anymore, the hall where there are no more fighting or memorable reconciliations, the silence that replaces the doors. I think about your life that now floats around you when you scream at the table, I think about you, I can't write: "I think about your son" singular, but I think about him too, your eldest, your son no, I can't write it, but I think about you two with the table facing each other. I think about the words that flew away, about the simple daily words that you can't pronounce anymore:

"Dinner's ready, boys," "bedtime, boys," "my sons," "my children," "the little ones," "the big one and the small one," "your brother," these words resonate so loudly when the others don't.

I don't know anything about your pain: I am like the child who observes the sky and sees only the planets that are burning, the stars in fusion. I don't know anything about your dead stars. I picture the apartment, but I forget the car, I erase those long trips that I never took, those trips through Paris under the rain, the freeway, the itineraries to imagine, try, the long rows of cars, the lights, and Sebastien sick on the seat. I avoid the anguish of time that passes by. The one of the brother who has to be alone, the hours of the day hospital 8h/23h, the pharmacy's hours, the prescriptions, I forget the medication bags, the paper folders that you had to take, the anuses and no parking spaces, the water bottles, the bathroom breaks, the cover when he was cold, the words you have to say to reassure in spite of the time, and the office where you didn't go this morning, the almost finished afternoon, and the pedestrians who continue crossing . . . The people should be told to look carefully, to the right and to the left, and pay attention to others. And the whole thing starts again, you come, you go, the hospital calls you back, he has to sleep at home tonight or maybe Thursday and "what day is today?" asks Sebastien.

Sometimes, it was not the same, with a lot of luck it was a hospital next to your house, sometimes it was another one, sometimes it was three times in the same week. I picture you in Paris with your red coat, your helmet and your gloves under your arms, your attentive look when the doctors talked with you, your smile to tell them that you were on their side, that you were courageous and that you were going to fight. I remember the scooter that you would always use in case of an emergency, I worried through email, but you wanted to join him as quickly as possible, you would always write to me after the facts, the scooter put away or abandoned, tied to a bench, a pole, a street light while you were bringing Seb back in a cab, while you were taking Seb in an ambulance, between life and death, to another service, to another hospital. I hear the emergency sirens that cross the city, on the back seat, I put my arms tighter around you to hold you when you come back alone, your hands clutched to the wheel.

You leave.

You're never home, always somewhere else, always gone.

You send me messages on my cell phone, some tenderness in 360 words and, most of the time, you're right on target.

You live every second intensely, since it seems unfair to waste any of this precious time that was taken away from Sebastien.

I call, I hear Sebastien's live voice on the answering machine where the three of you take turns saying your name. He's the last one to talk with a high pitched note, like a joyous conclusion: "and Sebastien!" I don't leave a message; I call back and listen a second time. You fly to the other end of the earth, you come back, you leave again. You need to "build another life, new memories" with your older son.

I protest, I worry about these extreme hikes in Africa where you try to lose your sadness, to scatter it, to distance yourself from it, to run faster and be ahead of it on another continent.

You don't try to forget, only to overcome the barriers of memories at the surface of your life, that always bring you back to a past where you drown.

It is said that during wars, soldiers who were sick would die on the front line, facing the danger.

You're walking in the grassy savanna, you sleep under the tent, you look for something that will kill a little bit of this pain that still burns inside you, overwhelms all your thoughts, tries to annihilate any attempt to live the present.

You read.

Remember this Saint-Exupéry sentence "the earth, he says, teaches us more than any book, because she resists us." You close the book and try to find some rest in the open night. Between you and the sky, only the material of the tent, somewhere, really close, the roar of lion, death with an exotic mask. Death, almost beautiful, dressed in its African mask. Death, simple, immediate, that kills in the present, the law of the jungle against which science is powerless, walks by you.

You fall asleep. You come back.

You show me pictures, a sky worthy of Hollywood when God spoke to Moses. A blue and yellow feel as if the sky had suddenly a center.

I smile and here he is, Seb, suddenly so close, with his tender look, his look that says "not a problem," when sickness had taken everything away, as if Saint-Exupéry had brought him back there on one of his night flights. With him, fragile lives, gazelles, their heads to the ground, zebras close to water ponds that look like clouds, a savanna in the sunset, blue birds with orange highlights, African babies who keep a fire burning. Life somewhere else more real, simpler, with the heavy skies that take you away from the light.

I spend the whole summer at the ocean.

I think about you, about him, non-stop. In the morning, when I look at the sky and while I get dressed, at night when the silence brings your voice to life. This morning, at the market, they were selling mother-of-pearl necklaces in heart shapes, and the little girls were buying them. I smile; it's delicate to protect a shell.

Tonight, in my room, at the feet of the chair, I find a trunk that you forgot, and in a corner, a pair of shoes resting on a Saint-Exupéry book, *The Little Prince*, of course, in a big format, as if you wanted me to join you in your race. As I opened the book, I saw an underlined sentence: "When the mystery is too overwhelming, you don't dare disobey."

I take a paper, intending to write to you. The first word that appears on the page is Sebastien. I write it, Sebastien, I make his name mine; I put it on paper to give him a body. Not a life, but a body because he is alive, in your apartment, in this house where I'm writing and he never came to, but that I had prepared for him, in your eyes when suddenly your look closes your jaw, in this seagull that was following us on this April morning as we were visiting the San Francisco Bay during this trip promised to Sebastien in America, in those planes that you keep taking. It's true that you travel a lot and that you walk, since you have time now.

A letter, just to tell you that I understand love and children.

One evening, at the end of the vacation, I read to you these pages. I open my laptop on the floor while you're lying on the bed, and I start talking. I tell you that I didn't have a choice writing these words, this book "Sebastien." I tell you that the words are difficult to tame. That I spent my days taking care of him like a mother takes care of her child, my nights talking to you. About things that we will never be able to fully express, as if words were always behind life, as if there was such a thing as unspeakable things, words that explode as soon as you try to write them on a page, as if they were round, at the same time heavy with emotions, pain and memories, but also light like the air, as light as the day when you're thinking about Sebastien watching little gray and white birds, jumping on the beach. On a brochure, their name in English: Godmarblethink, marble thought of God or small

marble, little ball with which God's thought play. Or I rather translate. Your heart to heart, your open heart, a little bit of you, a little bit of him, a little bit of me to bring back the bubbles on the page.
You cry a whole night in my arms.
You tell me a few words, correct a date, remind me of how it really was, take refuge in your hand caressing mine, the shared silence, and the sadness of the end of the summer.

The following day I go back to America, start writing to you again: small unimportant words in the present, uttered between two errands, breakfast that has to be prepared, the children that have to be taken to school, homework, my classes to prepare, the washing machine to start, the dishes to put away.
You don't answer right away, apologize, and tell me that everyday you write to me mentally, that you understand that it's not easy to read across the Atlantic, send me kisses. I wait for the evening to read you, write to you, and pick up the story. I wait for the night to steal your words, take them in my arms, unfold them one by one, untie them slowly, go look behind the petals of your courage, your modesty, your pain, the ink of your memory.

I meddle with your solitude. You tell me that you like the slowness of you writing to me.

It was the spring holidays in April 2000, you went to visit, with your two boys, the abbey of Thoronet, Sebastien has a cold, not really a sore throat, no exterior sign of the sickness, or weakness, but lumps, "lups" he would say as if he were talking about an enemy came from another planet or a cartoon.

On Monday, after a week's vacation at his grand-parents, you take him back to the doctor because the antibiotics didn't have any effect. He prescribes tests to be conducted first thing in the morning. Sebastien is suddenly tired "he can't stand up, I had to carry him," you tell me to make me under-stand the sudden weight that has invaded him. You fear mononucleosis. I try to reassure you. At the lab, in the afternoon, they don't want to give you the results, you're surprised, and they call the di-rector who confirms: the results will be given to the doctor. Already the worry, the time of a few seconds that hesitates. But the present calls you back, like a broken road that asks for your atten-tion. Your eldest goes on a school trip to Manches-ter, you're in a meeting at the school when your cell rings. It's the doctor who tells you that Sebastien needs to go back to Necker Hospital for new tests, then calls you back because there's no

room, which makes you smile because Necker, you were just thinking about it, "don't exaggerate."
You don't know yet that Sebastien has an allocated room, at the other end of Paris, at Trousseau Hospital.

He might already know it when, exhausted, sick in the cab that takes you away, he asks if it's still far. At Trousseau you have an appointment on a strange floor where children are bold. You can't imagine that you're in the right place. You still think about the lack of room in Parisian hospitals and you're sure that it's not really smart.

A whole team is waiting for him, takes care of him, plugs wires into him. You're thankful that he's well taken care of, impressed by the staff and the material used.

His dad calls; you can't talk because they tell you that cells are forbidden. You feel like you landed in a strange land with even stranger laws you don't know.

It lasts for a long time, a few hours, until you understand that they won't let you go: the child is now tied to drip wires that are attached to an electric pump in the wall. You feel trapped, behind an iron curtain you were not expecting, robbed of everything, of changing clothes, food, taken by surprise with only a purse to spend the night here. You tell Ariane who shows up for back up, bringing you a little support and food.

In the evening, the child falls asleep in the hospital. You don't take your eyes off of him, you stay by his side, you wait and the hours go by. You draw around him a space of silence; you look at his peaceful face, in his breathing something that will reassure you, something that will contradict the hospital. You protect him from the people who come and go, from the machine's noise, from the blinking signals, you would like to understand, you're conscious of your life suddenly thrown on an unknown road, at full speed.

You call a friend doctor with the tests results. She can't answer you right away. Silence. And then she cries on the phone, tells you a gray story of courage about an illness that lasts a long time that lasts an indefinite amount of time. Long. Patience. Courage. These are words that come back.

In the night, you start realizing the road traveled: two days and it's the heart of a hospital. You get ready for the days to come: stay in the hospital, no weekend trips, no school, homework to catch up, your professional meetings rescheduled, a more complicated life only after a few days, maybe a few weeks. Explain all of this to Seb, who has already asked, "when do we leave?"

On Wednesday the doctors ask to talk to the parents. They say "the father and the mother of the child," as if it they were common nouns, as if it would protect them from the terrible words they have to pronounce, address them to the patient's parents, nobody in particular. Nobody. They say the exact name of the sickness "it's leukemia." You ask if it's a cancer, just to be sure that you heard the name right, like a door that shuts. They don't say that you can never cure it. They don't say that it can last five years: They say what you can hear on this day, with spring around the corner, your will to live, your short term projects, your little boy's impatience to run, who yesterday was still in perfect health.

They say six weeks.

It's the first step. You don't know that as soon as you have the strength, they will step beyond your level of tolerance to accommodate the sickness. You think you can win some time, you bear everything, hurry to step beyond what is asked of you so that you can reach quicker the next step. Sebastien shows the same courage, the same tenacity: "If as soon as you have a little fever you cry, it's going to be a tough ride" he sighs as he is scolding his little neighbor.

They say two months.

On Thursday, everybody is at the hospital, Sebastien is in a normal room for only two weeks. They explain to you how the department works, the hours, the visits, they introduce you to the dietitian, the social worker, and the nurses. Your new family.
And you don't want it, and you don't listen.
They talk to you in a weird language with new words, new measurements. The weather is not nice, it's not gray, and it's white or red, white and red blood cells. It's the weather that grows or that weakens, and every day you ask what the weather is going to be like. If the bad white stay, it will be the black clouds of the sickness, if there's no more red, it's an emergency, blood in a short term that gives him back a little energy and color on his cheeks, if there's no more blood cells the veins are fragile, the hemorrhage risks, the bruises on your whole body. The shattered pieces on your soul when you punch my hand now to show me: "You do this, you have a bruise."
You learn to live with this new language. It's a matter of life, a matter of time spent in the hospital, you don't think about death.

After two months, in May, his room is considered "sterile": a sign "isolation" is hung to the door to point to the sickness. Winter in the middle of spring. People walk in the hallway and read the sign. Behind the closed door, an isolated child who hopes for what is forbidden. A lonely child whose loneliness is protected.

The visits are limited. To go close to him, you now have to wear blouses, masks, wash your hands. Make the volatile colors of the light disappear. Become transparent. Everything that surrounds him becomes a danger. Everything, that means you too, you who gave him birth, who gave him this weak body, fragile, this body that you can't take back, exchange for yours. You can't have the slightest cold, your heart stops at the slightest sneeze.

They tell you that an isolated room has just been made available. They tell you that you're lucky, and your luck is that you now live in a building protected like a fortress with a bell, guard, and drastic hygiene measures. I picture Laurent, returning from his visits, telling me about the rituals, the special soaps, the hand washing up to the elbows, the surgical hat, the bag on the shoes and his efforts to make Sebastien laugh with his Smurf disguise. His fear, and yours to contaminate him.

Seb is on his bed like in an igloo on a glacier, in an endless night, with no firm ground. He talks about the outside, the streets and the countries that he would invent when he went here and there with his buddies, his nanny, hang out in the park, in the woods. You invent, for him , each day, the fire, the air, the earth and the water.

Dreams, sand or ice deserts that have to be disinfected. Toys, books, clothes that you have to wash, bring back to the hospital, promise while they are being sterilized.

Numerous desires.

You juggle with the time of the sickness and the child's impatience.

He asks for a toy. You look in the box on the floor, trying not to make anything fall. Everything that falls on the side is lost.

He hangs on to your movement of firm ground, he asks for sceneries, he desires pictures, planes, he draws, he needs his pastels and his notebook that fell down, a game that's not heavy, tiny, yes, the one in his bedroom, on the right. He explains it to you. The visible and the invisible, what is said and what is hidden behind his plastic animals. He occupies the space, the whole space of his life, huge and the bedroom is narrow.

Around him a slue of products that are supposed to protect him from the dust, from any kind of germs, from the wind that he can't hear anymore behind these plastic bandages. These are transparent, resembling those curtains that our grandmothers used to put in their kitchens as a protection against insects. Around him, inside the barrier, three people take turns, only three visits a day, carefully chosen, because fifteen minutes count as a visit.

Every day, being there for the look of his face.

Outside of the movement, the television, the video tapes in unlimited number, the impalpable source of a world that you bring to him.

Now and then, a fourth person comes to see him. She stays next to the television, doesn't have the right to go into the sphere. She accepts to stay far away, behind the plastic bands, the continuing hum of his breathing. She talks with a soft voice, with a voice that doesn't hear, she stares without seeing.

He shows his pale face to everyone.

The sickness makes him hungry, an endless hunger, with no hope of being satisfied, and it weighs on his stomach with all the weight of what's forbidden and the medications.

He defends himself as he can, repeats a hundred times a day the forbidden words, draws them: raclette,* ham, onions, pickles, more and more, raclette, ham, onions, pickles, like the curious refrain of a song that he asks us to sing and to repeat to him, that we promise for later, at the end of the war, when the time for salt will be back, even if it never comes back because there will never be cheese, ham, onions, pickles to quiet down this terrible void, unsatisfied.

He cries about it.

For you, outside of the bedroom, in the building, no way out. No dining room, no family room. A tender nudity with him that calms him down and drains you. Wanting to go pee is half an hour lost: you have to leave the room, then ring the bell again, wait for the door to open again, wash yourself again, disguise yourself. Walk backward, incredulous, exhausted.

You say "each week is two weeks ago. The week inside, the week outside."

* Brand of cheese

He says "six weeks in there."
You take my sheet of paper, you draw a rectangle, "it's the bed," next to it a square, "it's the night stand," on the other side another square, a "toilet seat" and "it was difficult to carry this little body on the seat without putting his feet on the floor," at the end of the bed the box of toys on the floor, bassinets, instruments to wash him, around, the curtain, beyond, the room. You don't say anything anymore. I pretend I'm writing so that you continue.

Sometimes his friends come to build him a sun from outside. Very rarely. His naked body has a hard time resisting the flames of childhood and the risk of infection is too high.
You regulate the visits, close the doors of his house of life. He doesn't protest, doesn't ask for any other news than, deprived from everything, being loved from you, his family, from Guillaume his brother, Pierre and Bertille, his girlfriend. The others telephone. The teacher too organizes the phone calls, not to tire him, creates a chain. But the phone doesn't work well, the front desk erases the calls, puts them through late. He doesn't wait for them anymore, he draws.
One day you show me his sketchbook, you go

through it with me. Inside, Laurent's stories of Africa, lions, waterfalls, drawings of his childhood nanny, flowers from Mauritius Island, houses, churches, villages in the sun and everywhere his signature with the date.

You remember the letters he received, wanted to read and reread and that we had to run through to destroy the germs before entering them under the sterile area. The drawings that we hung on a poster board outside, next to his bed, the pictures of the desert, the soccer players, the drawings where he dreamt about food, prepared recipes, this magnificent illustrated letter that he wrote to your sister Catherine to thank her for having invited him to sleep over in a bedroom that she had specially prepared, all clean, like a dream that you talk about, in her house, in the outskirts, when he came out of isolation.

"Parents tell us things that don't make us laugh." He's tired of being there, he has used all the time and space of the bedroom. We try to link him to the outside with a computer equipped with a camera. But he wants the freedom of the light, he can't stand the image of himself without hair, the mess of being on a bed, the way others look at him, the space narrowed by the presence of the screen in front of him. We take the computer away.

He invents stories, men, plants, free animals, who run around in his room in spite of the sickness' branches, who come closer, stay at the feet of his bed, surround him, protect him, "The others don't understand what it's like to stay like this all day long." He doesn't read his buddies' notes anymore, he lives in the room that doesn't have windows. The crazy room. This room that nobody can understand. Nobody.

And the six weeks go by.
Time finally allows opening the doors of the new-found childhood. It's a joy to say the 29th of May: the sickness has been stopped, he can go out, celebrate his birthday.
10 years old, the 2nd of June.

Triumphant return in your car, washed, like new, looking 10 years younger. You laugh in the clean new car, eating a jar of pickles with the doctor who takes care of him.

You want to celebrate, the summer of his release,

make it a memory. Organize a giant raclette. You plan on inviting his friends, your family, and his classmates. You imagine partying worthy of your little ten-year-old prince, of his courage, a party that pushes away the night that erases the sickness. They remind you what the rules are.

The fight is not over, there's no resting, never, not at home, not anywhere, and he brings the sickness with him. You have to help him, no more than five people in his presence, chase away the tired people, chase away the dust, avoid the stuffed animals, take off the shoes walking into the apartment, manage strictly the refrigerator keep nothing beyond 24 hours, no fancy meals, no salt, follow daily the dietitian's advice. Explain all of this to Yasmine, his childhood nanny who makes sure that the household is well taken care of, like when he was a newborn.

You now buy vegetables, cellophane wrapped products, tiny portions that he starts, that you throw away, that you sometimes finish. You eat with your older son the leftovers, you shop all the time, add the stores' hours to the hospital's hours and the pharmacy's hours. For the first time in your life, you cook. You pay attention to the cooking utensils, to low fat cooking, to steamed cooking, to the cooking that makes the meat juicy, you buy a table, a table cloth, chairs. You buy furniture, drawers for the kitchen, for his bedroom, a bed because he can't reach his bunk bed anymore. You organize the apartment, you get rid of the trinkets, and you're cleaning all the time.

It will be long, but the results are good, he doesn't need to go to the hospital anymore, he can be nursed during the day.

The doctors say eight months.

You ask for a day surgery at the Ambroise Paré Hospital, closer to home. They agree but the Trousseau Hospital remains his main hospital, the cradle of his sickness, a necessary evil now and then. "At each step," he summarizes, like on his game boy.

You become the relay of his medical files. The schedule is simple: in the morning, tests, in the afternoon the treatment. Examine, wait, decide if there should be blood or if the treatment can be done, inject products one after the other, eliminate, multiply, feed, destroy, go home. Be able to come back to start all over again. Departure in the morning around 7 o'clock, return at night, sometimes at 11 o'clock. Go by the admission office in case of an emergency; go back to the admission office on the way out. Hours of waiting, hours wasted, hours during which you are both separated as you are filling in files, hours during which he waits in halls with drafts. You organize yourself twice as much, you prepare a dossier with all the necessary papers for a quick admission. You're on time at all your meetings with Sebastien, late with the administration who keeps asking you for papers they haven't received, papers you didn't send back on time.

For a test not done, a treatment started too late, he sleeps in the hospital or has to come back the next morning. You learn how to detect the traps, you predict numbers the day before, in a laboratory next to you, and at home to avoid the waiting rooms and the proximity of sick people, you try to win some time for treatments in the morning, you fight to minimize the moments when he is in the hospital, multiply the ones when he's in the softness of his home. You now know the time it takes for a blood transfusion, the effects that each product has on him. You make sure that he can escape, for a lunch at Mamita's, for a walk. You learn by heart the medications, the notices, the interactions, and the secondary effects to better understand the prescriptions. For each day, such or such pill, to take before or after a meal. For the medication prescribed in the hospital that you don't find in a pharmacy, for a cramp, nausea, you don't panic anymore.

On your agenda, hospital, hospital. Non-stop. Laughing, you say: "In July I worked, look at all these meetings, I worked, I had a great time." I think, "for once I was here," with this wound , like a splinter that I still have, for being absent, first bedridden, then expatriated.

The first time I came to see him in the hospital, it was in July, I could barely walk.

"Well!" he said as I walked through the door, "it takes a really long time when you break your leg!" I slipped on ice, in March. He got sick about ten days later, a simple sore throat, nothing serious, swollen glands, leukemia, everything went so fast, like my left ski on the snow.

We both stay a few days, sometimes at the hospital, sometimes at home, both unable to walk, clumsy, diminished. My crutches, him and his cap, both tired. We make a bet: the first one to heal, the first one who is able to run.

When he's allowed to go out, we go in the little park at the edge of your building, we sit on a bench, after dangerously going down the six floors. We are both out of breath. We stop at the same place. He's afraid he will have to go to the bathroom, I reassure him, I'm afraid I won't be able to go back up. He gives me his hand, tells me that he will help me . . .

I tell him that our bench is a boat, both of us on the boat, and the others far away, those who play in the sand box-germ box, those who work in offices as we are sailing on the ocean, those who are wasting their time in traffic when the fishing is miraculous . . .

I'm interrupted by the arrival of a young girl who comes next to us: she wants to ask us a few questions for a survey. She asks us what kind of facilities we would like in the neighborhood, he answers for both of us, "some sun, a lot more sun" because it has started raining and, all serious, he adds that he is sick, that it doesn't show but that it is a very serious sickness, and as she looks embarrassed, he says: "but it's not too serious."

Another day, he talks to me about his girl friends, he finds them pretty. He tells me what his taste in women is, looks at me, examines my dress, I'm wearing a blue dress, elegant, feminine shoes and a cast: "you're very classy;" I was supposed to go to a party, he was supposed to spend the weekend at his dad's, but his levels didn't raise enough, "insufficient levels," we both stayed in the light of the room, alone like at about the top of a lighthouse, it's the title of a documentary that talks about the ocean. I tell him that we are the last guardians of the hospital. He can't stop talking, he describes to me women who are wearing tight pants, lace underwear, yes, he knows about it, and "they must really itch," women who color their hair, in red, in orange. He gives me examples, holding my hand. He tells me that I am his type, like his cousin who is so pretty with her long hair, he wants me to tell him about his past, about his dad, he puts the families back together, he asks me to tell him again about Poland in a carriage, and how cute he was with his blond curly hair, how obnoxious he was screaming as a baby when he would wake up the whole house, he begs me to sing the love songs from before the war, the songs that my mother used to sing to me. He tells me that he feels good, falls asleep in the dim light of the bedroom, the curious rhythm of the machines and the sound of my voice. I come back in the morning, I buy cream in a nearby pharmacy. The pharmacist sells it to me with a lot of sweetness, he tells me that it's difficult to go to the hospital on this beautiful day, that the cream is light, that it hydrates the skin "like a fresh bath in pure water." I bring back the miraculous cream, the one that takes all the fears away, like all the pains. Seb is easy going. He gives me his body without restrictions. I wash him, the cream, change his T-shirt, his boxers. A little boy, all clean. We're proud of ourselves. He thanks me, tells me that it felt good and that I have soft hands. The next day, I start again, the cream is our alibi for the tenderness I give him and he receives and accepts.

I stay a few days, and I have to leave, I have to leave Paris, meet with my children in the South of France. I promise vacations, soon, a month, sweetheart, a month and you'll see, in August with Pierre. I promise fishing trips, I calculate the time, the days we have with Laurent to put together this house we just bought, empty the boxes, clean, buy sheets, make the beds. I give the recipe for fish soup, I explain the type of fish, their living patterns, and the fishing pole already bought by Pierre and prepared for him.

I kiss him, showing him my hand. It's agreed for 30 days. And after, you know, you will visit America, get well soon sweetheart, heal so you can come see the Pacific Ocean.

Mamita takes my place that morning at the hospital when I leave, when I don't know that it's the last time, that's why I try to leave quickly, I don't want to make him feel sad, that's why it takes so long to walk through the hallways today, walk past the door, go down the stairs, go out of the hospital with this sigh, so loud that a young woman who was sitting in the outside hall smoking a cigarette turned around.

Deep inside me, I sigh, I can't exhale, the weight of this last time, the beige raincoat that his grandmother was wearing, the kiss that she gave me as I was not leaving, the smell of her perfume and Sebastien's smile, happy to have both of us, showing the game I had just given him. I remember he said to me that he was lucky, that Mamita looked at me because we both shared the knowledge of a little boy that a sickness could not bring down.

I left Sebastien, and we both had dinner, on Buci Street. You wanted to take me to the restaurant, before I left Paris, take me on your scooter, because I couldn't walk. We saw the Luxembourg and pictures of "the earth seen from the sky." I was afraid to fall, I was holding you by the waist. I had bought books, homework notebooks for Sebastien, you had bought, to please me, lemon pies that we were supposed to eat together. We stayed late, I forgot the books and you forgot the pies.

You write to me today that you ate the pie that was intended for me, thinking about me with each bite, that you were laughing as you were swallowing, that you were not hungry, that you only ate it because you couldn't throw it away.

Beginning of August, your family goes on vacation.

You hope to leave Paris to come to the South of France with your two children. The hospital in Toulouse has agreed to ensure the follow-up of the treatment, but the doctor hesitates. It's difficult to set up, to plan. The child waits. To everybody, he gives his patience, his trust. The doctor calls, gets the meetings, the authorizations.
A departure is possible after a last treatment at Ambroise Pare.
You think. The issue of transportation is almost impossible to resolve. The plane is forbidden, and you can't really jump over the Loire. You organize a car ride, buy a CD player, and look at the maps. Ten hours. It's impossible. You negotiate, manage to convince the hospital that a one hour plane ride is better than a ten hour car ride, you insist: On Monday, there are very few people on the plane.
The medical team gives the OK on Friday afternoon.

I wait for you; I write your arrival time on a notepad next to the telephone that gives me a friendly look, each time I walk through the room. Laurent and I are on schedule, the beds are made, the house is clean, and the fishing pole is ready.

And suddenly on Saturday, the sickness comes back with an amazing violence, wild, that doesn't want that vacation. Sebastien screams with pain, calls for help without you knowing how to relieve him, without you knowing if you have to take him to the hospital on this 14th of August.

You call, you don't get an immediate answer, you jump in your car with your two boys, drive on the shoulder in the emergency of your distress.

Sebastien slowly calms down. He loves when you drive fast. It's what he tells you a little later.

You call me, an avalanche of pain in his body, naked, away from all treatment. He has a fever, the doctors don't understand why. They have to open, operate without waiting any longer. Sunday August 15th.

I remain speechless on the phone.

We don't have any more dreams in stock, no tropics, no snow to make you feel better; we have nothing to offer in exchange.

You stay in a very hot Paris, behind glass doors that maintain a surreal temperature, unbearable. You're alone, Paris is on vacation. I stay in the South of France, in a useless house, motionless, on the eve of a move to America. Pierre goes fishing, with a stain of silence on his forehead.

Sebastien is the first who starts living again.

He is locked in his bedroom, with his imaginary changing skies, the rivers as long as hair, the clothes matching the garden, the sea, the trees that border the marshes. And he tells them to a friend, a child prisoner like him, lying at the foot of the machines. He is from Martinique, with the same sickness locked in his body. He likes to listen to Seb, his hidden voice that makes his nights shorter, the delicate movement of the trees, their height next to the sky that bend according to the wind, the rain, the sun.

The floor, the ceiling, the walls to which they are both attached, makes them inseparable. In the ward, they call them Dupont and Dupont, they talk, they play, never stay at the same place, they come and go from the marshes to the ocean, play endless games of game boy and Nintendo, organize water fights with needles, mix up the nurses' names with an innocent air, turn off their neighbors' televisions with the remote, end up getting scolded like children. They laugh.

You laugh too when you tell the stories and you're in awe on the phone.

End of August, you're given permission: four days in Normandy.

It is a strange vacation, busy, close to the fights. You organize water fights with raincoats and rain boots not to catch a cold. You take Seb to the seaside, a forbidden sea, but one that still moves and that he is permitted look at, to enjoy the immense happiness of listening to it, come and go, constantly on the beach, you take him to visit an abbey "what is roman style?" listen to the silence, run; become a child again, come out of the sickness to go crab and shrimp fishing, buy one more time a fish net for two hours, knowing that it might be the last time, and it was the last time, cut the flowers in the garden, go for a walk on the cliffs of Etretat, show your behind to say no to photographs, play Ping-Pong, eat bread on the pier at Honfleur since you're not allowed to go to restaurants, not allowed to eat any kind of food that's not under cellophane, find everything beautiful, put on Pitou's blazer, even if it's too big, rest in the evening, in front of the fireplace in the middle of summer. Crack up laughing at the hospital, thinking about the door that you had forgotten to open in the fireplace, about the cloud of smoke that you had to walk through, in order to go to the kitchen to fill in the plates with spaghetti, about the pharmacy bag used to put the shells.

Today you show me the pictures of these four days that lasted so long. A picture of Sebastien at the foot of Victor Hugo's statue built where Leopoldine drowned "poor Victor Hugo." It's random, you say. Other pictures follow, an abbey, cows, shadowy and lit pictures with a stormy sky on one side, a blue sky on the other. "It's at the same place," you add.

September comes. The chemotherapy continues. The end of the treatment is planned for February, in the middle of the school year. You try to plan the future, establish certificates in a record time, fill in forms, and get a school support system at home through an organization. You have to find a volunteer. In his school.

Because there is a school: On the eve of the first day of school, surprise, they tell you that he's coming out of the hospital, that he can go back to school, be there on the first day. You run to a su-permarket, at dusk, to buy him school supplies. There's nothing left, the sales people smile ironi-cally when you ask for a backpack and a pencil case. "There's nothing left, madam, it's a little bit late!" The next day, you find this blue and yellow backpack that Pierre continues to wear and that he refused to give up last September. You want new clothes; you're looking for Mao collars, to match his bold head, little Tibetans clothes. In your agenda, there's still the yellow post-it with the store's address.

So he goes to school, on the first day, sits in class next to a little boy who gives him the strength to take off his cap under his teacher's look. He tries, as much as he can, to lead the life of a normal child. But the sickness looms, he is not allowed to run, to jump, and to rumble at recess. A security zone is set up around him in the schoolyard, to help him be good. He is allowed to bring cards, and small toys.

He is protected from falling, from the games that could tear the catheter, from any extreme tiredness, from all germs, the burning of the sun, the wind, the feeling of loneliness when he is in the heat of the classroom, the intense looks.

The enemy is everywhere.

It's vital to talk to the other children's parents to ask them for help: they have to be responsible, signal all sickness, every risk of contamination, say if their child has a cold so that yours stays at home.

You also have to calm them down, explain to them the sickness, reassure them because they're afraid of AIDS, of the contamination of pain, of destiny, of the tragedy of a sick child.

You take advantage of the beginning of the year meeting to talk, the sick child is yours: you look in the eyes of those who are listening to your speech, you the mother of a child with leukemia. Their curiosity, their compassion, their fears. Their ignorance of what your life is when you go home, alive, intact, in good health, with a body and legs that work, woman, mother, a healthy child and a sick child.

So he goes to school. He has a teacher who understands the absences, the late homework, the buddies' looks, the lack of balance between his life of a little boy and his life of a patient, the fears of getting bad grades and the fear of bad cells. She offers to be the volunteer to give him four hours of tutoring a week, tells him that he is a good student, that he is serious and that he will grow up.

He doesn't go to school anymore, but he is the best student in class. The best students tell him with a surprised air, but nobody is thinking about taking his place. He wants to please, avoid mistakes, writes his numbers as best as he can when he's doing exercises. On the bulletin board, good grades and great teachers' comments that deliver him from the present, throw him in a future where his children will be proud of him. Sometimes, the sickness is too strong; the sickness jumps over the homework and takes over the white pages of his notebooks. Two hours saved of school this week. None the following week, none the one after that. The notebooks stay in the backpack.

His teacher comes to visit him in the hospital. She finds him weak, it's written in his eyes, he tries to console her, gives her a dinosaur for her little boy, shows her family pictures, wedding pictures, tells her about the joy of eating pizza tomorrow and taking baths.

He's getting used to his new life, "you get used to it, I was taught," bad cells and blood cells weakening, it's the sickness that goes back but it's also the tiredness, the exhaustion, the organism, emptied of all substance until the levels go back up, when the sickness disappears, the time of a remission of a few days, and it's the following treatment.

Very few days when he feels good.

On his nightstand, drawings of children, letters from his classmates, with a note from his teacher, the one before, from sixth grade. He remembers her, she used to scold him a little bit, when he sang while he was working because "you see, she would say: it's not the time but she was happy because we were happy." It's with her that he went skiing last year, it's she who asked for tights to put under the pants, but "it's not necessary because I was not cold, I didn't even fall." In a letter, she wrote "my little man," he smiles he thinks that he's not that small, that teachers are like mothers, that they can't help giving us funny names: sweetheart, kitten, sugar. Well "little man" he sighs: "it's not that bad." At the hospital, you organize the visits, you prepare everything according to the number of people who are allowed in his room, the ones he really wants to see, the ones who are available, you phone, give away schedules, leave messages.

Your mother fills in for you.

The whole family jumps in, I didn't know your sisters, Pitou the little one, his beloved godmother, Catherine the big one. They look like you: the same determination, same smile came from outside, still full of Paris' rain, the bridges on the Seine, the passersby and "do you know Seb what I saw on my way here? A dog all wet, so wet, Japanese children, yellow leaves still hanging on to the trees, a yellow cab like in the United States," the same kisses, the same amount of time given without counting, the same words full of light that resonate, constantly on the telephone.

At the beginning, he doesn't like to use it, intimidated by the echo of his voice, by the silence, the necessity to say something, with definitive words that you can't catch up, can't correct with a look. Very quickly he learns how to use it, send messages, answer, with a slightly serious movement when he grabs the phone that shows the amazement he feels, bedridden and using a phone. Very quickly, he knows how to tame it, talk, but also have conversations, connect with his childhood voice, impatient, endless of dreams and present that amaze him.

As soon as he comes home, you throw a party: on pictures there are children in socks, children barefoot, children around a table who share a meal. A raclette, you say, he would dream about one every time he went into the hospital, couldn't stand the children who played with the food on their plates.

In the fall, there's his cousin's wedding.

Up to the previous day, he dreams about it. He looks very closely at the monitors, orders the levels to stay low. "Please, please." The levels obey him: he's very tired but can go out. During the party, you verify the dishes, control what he's eating, and bring him surprises in individual packages so that he's not disappointed.

He becomes a little boy again, plays soccer, and wants to go boating at nightfall, sleep with the others in the dorm. You bring him to the hotel with you to sleep.

It's in October that it happens. Suddenly. The invasion.

He starts trembling, has a lot of fever, his right arm doesn't respond.

The professor, who heads the hospital service, examines him. In spite of the terrible crisis, the spasms, the convulsions, in the heart of the storm, he gives the impression that he's managing the situation, that he has Sebastien's body under control, that he knows where he's going.

But Seb has lost his body's integrity: a part of him is dying. After the arm, the leg, the whole right side has a problem, doesn't respond to him anymore. He's now dependent on others, can't stand up, walk, pee, get dressed, and play. He can't talk, articulates the sounds that his mouth refuses to produce.

He cries because he's afraid of being paralyzed.

He has crises every day.

He can't say that he's afraid anymore.

Sometimes the crises are so violent that they have to put bars around his bed, to attach him. It's what he says with a veil of sadness that translates his lack of power to calm the waves of hurt in his body: "I was tied." "Sometimes, you're tied."

You talk about the nurse; you say how relieved you

are to know that she is by his side in these cell wars, star wars. She goes to see him all the time, explaining to him the fight in his body as if it were a ship. He listens with an infinite patience.

With you, no, he doesn't have any patience; he waits for you to understand with the eyes.

The crises come in succession.
They take the child, they look, make big circles in the water of the sickness. They are numerous, getting busy around him: the stretcher-bearers, the nurses, and the doctors, on the other side of the doors that are closing. And nothing. It's what they come to tell you: "nothing." They don't know what's going on in the mystery of his body.
They don't try to explain it to you.
You don't ask any questions.
Powerless.
Them.
You.
They still go for it, persevere, perform several lumbar punctures.
The verdict is in: "Complication: early deterioration." Early deterioration because he was in remission. Early because it was the middle of the

treatment. Now the sickness is in his brain.

But you don't understand anymore.
You did, with Sebastien, two of the four pages that were in the protocol. Eight months, the doctors had said, and now they don't say anything after the word complication. Now, after all these months of climbing, the summit has moved out of your reach. You were counting the number of lumbar punctures remaining and there's no ending in sight. In three days, he just had two.

"As he is breathing the anesthetic product," you explain, "he recites, non stop, for fifteen minutes, half conscious, mom, and the name of his brother and Pierre's name." It's what you describe to me, his love for Pierre to avoid the beginning of the shock treatment that he has just been prescribed, as if what he had gone through these last months had been for nothing.

It's at that moment that you stop working a few days.

The doctors just admitted that the treatment is not enough anymore, that they have to try a transplant. For the first time, you have doubts; you realize that they're failing.

You call people at night; you go to the other end of

Paris, in the suburbs to talk about unconventional medicine. That's all you do, you don't trust medicine anymore. Seb and you had agreed to everything, and that everything was not enough. The feeling that you had dealt with things beyond your limit and the sickness is still here, victorious. So you say: "They don't know, it's not possible."

When you talk about it, you are told that conventional medicine and alternative medicine can't co-exist, they tell you about scientific fights, an economic war, political. But, you write, "a parent doesn't care about all of that when his child is sick! He doesn't understand why they don't do EVERY-THING humanly possible, everything that has been proven on both sides, and why not shark oil, if it works!! If it helps, even a little bit!!"

The sickness doesn't care about your mindset, your weariness, it continues its work. One day, Seb falls on the stairs, his brother calls the firemen, calls his grandmother for help, another day he has violent cramps as soon as he comes out of the hospital.

The episodes come in succession, always dramatic, always violent, with, each time, the fear of a trauma for life, definite lesions. One day, Seb can't get his body to function again, another his right eye takes a long time getting back to normal. They're so small, so little the blood vessels when you think about it, so easy to lose command of the brain.

You try to reason, and there's no reason why you shouldn't be afraid.

The doctors try to understand.

They put him under completely to look for the sickness.

But the roots are deep, the trip is too long and the child doesn't come back to the surface. Panic, he doesn't have any more heart rate or blood pressure. "It's not true." That's what you must be thinking.

A doctor tells you that his brain is maybe damaged. They decide to transfer him to Necker Hospital, neurosurgery service, nine at night. You bring his stuff, bring the food, a change of clothes. Impression of a perpetual transit. In the meantime, he wakes up. You follow the ambulance on a scooter. You park.

He's not in neurosurgery, but in the resuscitation ward. Too late, the door closes: visits end at eight o'clock.

They ask you to go to the admission office to open a file.

It's the procedure.

For him too.

For every patient brought in an emergency.

A year in the hospital doesn't change anything.

He's on the other side, behind the glass door, alone.

It's the rule.

You know what is asked of you, because without

the "labels" that have a file number, they can't do any tests.

You discuss; explain that neither you nor he were aware of a transfer in a forbidden zone.

You manage to cross the demarcation line, find him in tears in an empty room, without anything in it.

A room without anything, only a bed and him on top, naked, not even wearing underwear.

Under observation.

In jail.

You warm him with your presence; they find him a soup and then two. You blow on his life, you keep the flame alive, the thirst to live in his veins, and you seem to be the only one who knows that he has leukemia, always, in spite of the resuscitation. You close the doors, and leave him once he's asleep.

The next day, you stay at his side, hiding, in this room without light or windows where visits are forbidden, leaving as soon as the visiting hours assure you that you can come back, trying to meet with the doctors who examined him in the morning, to find out more. After endless hours of waiting, you find them, question them.

The same word comes back, always the same: "his state is back to normal, the sickness is hiding," somewhere far away. They're thinking about an

expedition, more tests, in the coming days, probably next week, somewhere else, maybe in another
hospital. But for now "nothing," a horizon empty
like a black mark that runs across the sky.

You refuse to stay there, in front of this motionless
ocean, in this blockhaus if you don't really have
to. You pick up the fight, make calls, and try to get
him out before the fateful date of the weekend.

You succeed. He stays only one day. He comes out,
goes back in the middle of the night to the Trousseau Hospital. The joy of simply being in a room.

You hang in there, you start your rounds again, and
him the invisible battles, somewhere, far, in this
silent war. More of a guerrilla, with unexpected
falls, a fight that makes no sense and that has no
end, with the fear of a predicted paralysis.

That repeats itself. Non-stop.

He comes out, goes back in. Complications tied to
the total lack of his immune system, the conse-
quence of the treatment that he has just endured.
He has fever, stays a week in the Ambroise Pare
Hospital.

You are disoriented. Leukemia here is not the same
as in Trousseau, you worry about the air, and the
germs, and you make sure that the doors are
closed. Things that have been kept away from him
for months, against which you were warned, sud-

denly are permitted. You forbid bread that stayed in the neighboring room, croissants that a nurse, full of good intentions, offered him. You feel like the last rampart before the sickness.

It moves forward, looks for your slightest sign of weakness, puts doubt in your soul, accuses you of keeping food away from him when he's so thin, and you don't know if you're right anymore.

November 12th, you write to me.

"Seb is still in the hospital. He just spent a week at Ambroise Pare and they couldn't bring his fever down. He has been in profound pain for ten days now. He will be transferred to Trousseau tomorrow . . . I'm sick and tired!!! (and him too!!!). All these hospital days, for nothing, not even to get better, without knowing how we're going to cure him in the months to come . . . A month ago, there were only four months to hang in there . . . STOOOOOOOOOOOOOOOOOOOOPPPPPPPPPPPPPPPP!!!! I stop. The hospital just called. They transfer him, in emergency, to Trousseau, there, now, right away . . . By the way, I have made a lot of effort in 2000 to stay Zen!!!

I so want to talk to you

Kisses

I run."

When you join him, Sebastien is sitting down, smiling; on a stretcher, in the hall, his body offered, calm, he's eating cookies waiting for the ambulance. A tension problem. He talks about his deregulated life, his ambulance adventure, is so happy about the siren and the light, welcomes you aboard his smile.

You arrive in Trousseau with him. Emergency service, they make you fill in papers, suddenly they ask you for your divorce judgment. You don't argue, you promise everything for the next day knowing that everything has been in his file for months. Being indignant, protesting doesn't serve any purpose, Sebastien is right; don't slide towards the obscure universe, the harsh words. You go back to him.

The present for now reduces itself to the abandon of his body to the machines that substitute for his vital functions.

He is asked to be a pure spirit, to step out of his skin, to trust the medical team, including for basic needs such as eating or peeing. And he does it, he positions himself on the bed and he takes off his body. Cold everywhere. Night comes, obscurity, no more human warmth, the emergency of the resuscitation services where only the fight against death matters, the sudden death, short term, with the body plugged to machines, their sound is at the maximum so that it can be heard at the other end of the hall.

They don't ask him anything anymore, they don't look at him, they observe the machines, they pay attention to the indicators they are transmitting, they examine the tests and they try to balance his levels towards the norm, towards life. No machine is supposed to be the speaker of his pain, of his fear, of his conscience jailed by his body.

Only you remain. You know that he's not an injured child. For him, the state of emergency, the restrictions, the exile from the house have been reality for months, years in his world, he's at the end of his rope, doesn't have any more strength.

You would like to take him by the hand, but you can't touch him, bring him comfort, the wires, the machines, everything keeps you away. You come closer to the legs, since the upper body parts are inaccessible, you caress the top of a foot, and on the other is a lozenge, a light that blinks.

Death is everywhere, she's waiting for him there, but there is just an adventure, an episode, death threatens him in the distance, over there, hiding in the ditches, the maze of his body.

You prepare him for the battles to come. You obtain a television, show him books on the adventure of writing that you have with you because of a project that you're working on. He draws hieroglyphics, Chinese symbols. He writes your name and his, love notes, darkens the pages, applies himself, and concentrates, under the admiring eye of the nurses. He reads the words aloud, follows them with his finger, brings to life the magical words, like the Pharaohs in the Pyramids' text: "the sky rejoices at your approach, it takes you in its arms, it kisses you, it caresses you; it puts you at the top of the glorified, the eternal stars."

At the bottom of a little bit of sun, lie today the days of resuscitation. Only the crystal of his softness remains in this thesis on writing that you are finishing this year and the simplicity with which he asked the nurses not to hurry his grandmother too much, when she came to visit him as if he was being finally "unplugged," to transfer him, at "home," at the hematology department.

Despite the difficult days and nights, he stays kind, considerate; he is the very sweet and very nice guardian of the fragile fire of his heart in the depth of the hospital.

In November, you are told that neither you, nor his father or his brother is compatible for the transplant. None of you can be a donor.

You bring him to the seaside. It's raining, you eat sandwiches in the car with a whole jar of pickles, he walks on the beach, can barely walk, pretends to run, mimes a fight with his brother, just enough time for a picture.

Beginning of December, still no compatibility in the donors' banks, it's an emergency, they plan on a transplant with the blood of an umbilical cord. They give you the new program: radiations, in January, to get rid of the sickness that has settled in the brain and a transplant that will start with a total irradiation. "The transplant is a complete isolation for six weeks, two people allowed, the father and the mother only." Seb, this time, goes out of the room, he doesn't want to hear what comes next. What comes next is that he will be sterile and that his growth will be partially stopped. In case of a success, of course, that is not obvious. You understand an experimental stage, a high-risk surgery before and after. You don't know if the transplant is a chance or not.

Saint Louis Hospital, the anguish and the worries for hours. From his weakened body, thin, they take and inject his blood again in sufficient quantity to recuperate the cells that could be necessary for a second transplant, in case the first one fails.

It's Christmas, he comes out of the hospital between the 24th and the 26th of December, the exact dates when, on the other side of the world, Pierre breaks his arm and takes his place for two days. He fills himself with salmon and raclette, even though salt is still forbidden "because" he says to explain it "with salt you blow up very quickly and it takes a very long time to deflate." He calls himself "little fatty Buddha," he is serene; I mail him Star Wars toys and a picture of Pierre he collects immediately like "the most beautiful gift."

You tell me of the caress of his fingers on Pierre's picture, every night, this picture of Pierre that he would kiss before falling asleep.

After Christmas, they prep him. Since chemotherapy has not worked, they start the radiations. Impossible to go backward, the transplant is unavoidable. At the Saint Cloud Hospital, they mark on his skin, the exact place of the impacts. They are six of them taking exact measurements. More than four hours checking his skin. You tell him that they have to do it. He cries, making sure that he's not moving.

January, the happiest month. Every day, he leaves in an ambulance: "Come on, quick, pass the truck, put on your siren, come on, the small white, pass it!" At night, he sleeps in his bed, he's absent from the house only two or three hours at a time for radiation sessions that are not too long. He laughs, gets back to his childhood games on his bedroom's rug, and organizes car races.

Very quickly, he doesn't need anybody anymore, he leaves with the ambulance driver by himself, refuses to take the sickness seriously. He dresses as inspector Gadget to cover the scars of the battle, absent hair and damaged right eye, adds a red nose on his nose to perfect the comedy of the sickness. He becomes the star of the St. Cloud Hospital, more used to adult patients, makes the nurses laugh, goes everywhere with his plastic briefcase that contains toys, wrapped snacks and small bottles of water.

They radiate his spine and the cephalo-rachidian bulb. Once again, he loses all his hair, with the exception, this time, of a little tassel on the front and another one on his neck. His spine is burnt, they apply cream.

He doesn't care, he can't help but be happy. Actually, it's over; the radiation treatment is finished.

You call me, you know that the transplant frontier is near. You are going to be forty, you still don't know if you're going to celebrate. I don't know anything about the last wounds, the last battles. You told me details very recently. The horror of the resuscitation rooms, the slightest skin parcel that becomes the field of all pains, the body being defeated, that can't be appeased. I don't understand, I encourage you to continue the fight, to get out of the trenches to charge the enemy, I scold you, I persist and you show great patience to explain to me that no, maybe defeat.

Laurent decides to join you in Paris, he has a mission, he can move it forward, go and see you, give you some strength back, especially go the hospital, carry Seb again, his bag and the bed, if necessary the whole bed, the wires and the machines. Laurent says that the fight goes on, that you shouldn't lose hope. Pierre asks at the dinner table if children can die.

The date is set at Robert Debre for the transplant.

Last big party at home before the big shut in, you invite his buddies, you organize a memorable water fight with syringes in the park. You want him to leave for his bubble with images of happiness. You give him provisions of laughter for his trip.

The 15th, he goes into the hospital. Everything is evaluated for hours. Each specialist examines his own domain, excluding others, you remember the dentist who wanted suddenly to pull one of his teeth.

Before the transplant, the body has to be completely irradiated. The whole body, but with the exception of the parts that were irradiated in January. He is measured again and again: you have one meeting after another. His schedule is very busy. He doesn't have a lot of time left, manages to have lunch, one day, with his friend Bertille at home, talks to her on a cell phone to tell her where he is, comes back home in twelve minutes zigzagging in the ambulance on the beltway.

The transplant is near.

On a Thursday night, Sebastien doesn't come home and stays in the hospital. The following day, he doesn't follow the regular schedule, the doctors ask to speak to you, they ask that the father be present.

They say the impossible: the sickness took advantage of these few days to explode; the transplant is no longer possible. He has to be transferred to the Trousseau Hospital.

You ask for a night's rest to catch your breath, you promise to be, first thing in the morning, at Trousseau and you bring him home to offer him one night in his bed.
He doesn't talk, goes directly to his bedroom, doesn't ask for anything and takes refuge under his sheets. Delivered from the noise, the doctors, the nurses, the neon light, the wires that attach him to the wall, he hides without moving. You sit next to him, you chat, caress his hand under the sheets, you manage to make him come out, to bring him, and the both of you eat, sitting next to each other, on the big sofa in the living room. Then you take him in your arms and you both stay there, crouched in each other's arms in a moment of unforgettable tenderness that lasts a long time, conscious to have stolen these moments of eternity from the hospital and the sickness. He falls asleep against you and you carry him to his bed.

At the Trousseau Hospital, after 24 hours, the doctors tell you that he has only three days left. The tests are worse than when he came into the hospital last year. They prescribe a very heavy treatment, a treatment of last resort.

Coming out of the meeting with the doctor, your sister Pitou is there, your brother, your brother-in-law. You're the only one who knows, you don't say anything, you offer a moment of life, a game of baby foot, an hour of happiness as a family. You want to see him laugh, offer him some joy, up to the end of his life, until his last breath, because life is beautiful . . . so that he thinks so again and again . . .

So that he is comforted.

And Sebastien is amazing of life and happiness. You can't imagine that he is dying, like the doctors just told you.

That night you announce it to Mamita, because of the emergency to live each day that are about to come.

You sleep in the hospital.

Monday goes by, you watch each hour that goes by. He has a problem with his kidneys, can't urinate anymore.

But the body overcomes the obstacle, goes back to work.

The three days go by, the tests reveal absurd levels, he doesn't get up anymore, doesn't play, death is taking him away, but death stays soft. You accept it, you simply wish that he remained the same, discreet; you accompany him, sliding, bringing gifts.

One day he calls you, he only says two words: "you come" and in these words the emergency. With him, quick. You probably never received just an explicit message. Not an order, not a request, not a complaint or a scream. More like a howling, transformed with all the strength of his love for you in one sentence, in words pronounced distinctly, with frailty. Two words: "you come" because there's nothing else to do, because nobody else but you can appease his suffering.

You run, you don't waste any time reassuring him on the phone, you don't waste time with useless words. You go, you take him in your arms, you push back the wires, you make room to sit next to him on the bed and you stay like this, in a unique transparency where he is against you while you gently caress his head, his smooth skull where there's only a few hair left, a small tassel on his forehead that makes him look like a wise man, his arms going up far under his T-shirt, and you look at each other ready to cross the last frontier and the last trip.

But the days continue to flow. The end of February comes, it's your birthday, forty years old, Sebastien manages to buy you a rose, asking the nurses for money. He offers it to you, like in the thirties song, to be present at your party. You bring him a cake, his favorite, vanilla ice cream, meringue and strawberries that he eats with you, his brother, Mamita and a friend . . . two people at a time in the room. He wants the nurses to enjoy it too, and he keeps a piece for them. At night, you keep the flower next to you, you ask to have a picture taken of you and Sebastien the rose, Sebastien already present in your mind.

The next day, you celebrate your birthday with the family, he sends you those who come to visit. Nothing is real, nothing but the heart to respect. It's what he tells his cousin, talking about a bird that comes sometimes on the iron balcony of his window. "Sometimes, I dream that I am him, the bird outside, that I'm flying, I take a walk in the forest." Then he tells him to go away, to join you, he wants you to have people around you.

Laurent comes back from Paris; he brings back pictures where he is with Seb. He tells us about you,

about Sebastien's father, about Seb, about your love that will surpass everything.
On the pictures, nothing but the sickness.

And the days go by. He hangs in there for a week.
On a Wednesday, you offer him the castle he dreamt about, he gets up, he wants to take a shower, doesn't stand up, starts playing again.
The visits resume, "the world thinks about me," he says smiling.
But he is in a time escaped from the procession of time; he is the bird on the window, the bird that jumps on the edge as the weight of sickness gets heavier each day.

The following week goes by, the doctors, who talk about a transplant again, say it's a miracle.
Then another week.
On Monday, he is told that he will get out Thursday to rest at home, the home hospitalization system is set, he's happy.
On Tuesday, fever comes back, his going home will now happen the following Monday.
On Wednesday, he records the tape of his interview.
On Thursday, the fever goes up, his skin is covered with pimples.

On Friday, he experiences tremendous suffering, not a centimeter of skin is spared. Suffering.
On Saturday, you ask that he be given stronger medication.
On Sunday.

You would like to remember the words exchanged in those moments, call them, hug them, like rays of lights at a house entrance, in the summer. The nurse who called him "sweetheart" coming into the bedroom, was going out, coming back in until Sebastien asked her: "Hey! You know that I'm going to get a puncture, you're here to reassure me? Have you had a puncture before?"
Tell the doctor, who had the same name as you, to what extent his gentleness had been important for Sebastien. Thank her because she understood separated parents, the medication that had to be taken in each house, the dreams of vacation, and the desire of the big brother to sleep next to the small one. Because she had a fair voice, a voice that didn't complicate the sickness to explain the room, to live and to fight, a voice that didn't lie to say that the fight would be long, months, maybe years. Because she was happy, because she loved life. Thank her for this permission given in August:

these vacations at the ocean, in Normandy in the little house lent by Ariane.

And there is all the others, the whole team of the Trousseau Hospital that nobody will ever take in their arms to tell them that it's not their fault if the sickness is the strongest, if life gets away from them sometimes, tell them to keep moving forward, show the way. A path of patience when the parents don't want to listen, when the children are too young and cry at night, that they have to have a transfusion, surgery, a transplant, in the desert of suffering, the suffering of the parents, alone in their homes that's not home anymore since the child is missing; the suffering of the children, alone in their body, flat on the mattresses, prisoners of the suffering that is transported, that is transferred, that is being rolled on beds, carts, that is taken in arms sometimes, and you have to take everything, the child and the suffering, pretending that it's not contagious, that it slides on the white blouses, blue, as if it were easy to see a being suffer, regardless of his age or life story. A path of courage when you have to tell the truth and the truth is the bottom of their heart that breaks, their heart that breaks endlessly, today and again tomorrow, because every day children get sick, every day they have to tell parents, explain to them the hospital, the fight, the weapons, the obstacles, talk to them about the danger, the strategies to adopt, without anything to help them convince, congratulate them, tell them that it's right, this path of courage of endurance even if they can save only one. A child and he's worth every one of them. And there is still pain. Because the child stays a child, in a suffering that nothing appeases, not even suffering.

He is never vanquished, until the end he exists with his naïve look, his child's words that the hospital walls can't stop, his amazing smile, his arms that he throws around his mother's neck, his grand-mother Mamita, his love for life. Up to the end, he forgives the suffering for being so crazy, for being born, for being here. And he is so handsome when he manages to run, play soccer one last time, illu-minate his cousin's wedding in September. It's a miracle to be a child, to be so happy about the married couple's happiness, of the family picture: "Can you imagine, Mamita, that it's thanks to you that there's all of this?" to be able to be there on that day, to be comforted about everything look-ing at them from the mezzanine. He doesn't need much, so little: a movie that he watches on televi-sion with his grandfather is enough for him to laugh, without hesitation. His laughter is such a marvel, coming from the river of the body that we thought empty, without any resources. And life is still there; "Tea for two" in "La Grande Vadrouille" and it's endless laughter that makes him forget the sickness, the cares that we have to take with this body so thin that it's transparent, such a laughter that the nurse comes. She stays a few minutes; it's enough for him to fall asleep. The movie continues, he will never know that Bourvil ends up in the beautiful girl's arms, but it's not finished, he's still laughing, at his worst, in the resuscitation room, where nobody watches television. For him, the rules were forgotten, and the TV is there, it doesn't work well, you can barely hear it and the image is bad. He doesn't complain, he doesn't say anything, subjected everything, silent. And when everybody thinks he's sliding, when all the machines have been asking for help, in vain, for a long time since they tried everything, suddenly a burst of laughter breaks out and shakes his whole body while, on the screen, a reporter, in the funniest outtakes, gets knocked over by a wave, at the seaside.

It's barely imaginable, a child. He persists, against all odds, to be, to move towards life, to like candies, for him it was the blue smurfs, five a day the doctors said "not one more and the open package has to be thrown away after 24 hours." "Great" he would answer because he could offer some to everybody who visited him, and the doctors, the nurses, the nurses' assistants, the tutors that he would fire since he had his private teacher.

He doesn't try to hoard things, he is given things and he takes them in the nest of his bed. He sits cross-legged and opens his hands: one day there are appetizer cookies, salty cookies that are forbidden, another day it's cheese that is sometimes allowed and that he loves, another day it's peach jam in small containers, canned pineapple. It's not easy to dampen the spirit of a child, he gets up at night, stretches the perfusion wire at his maximum and goes to see the little girl they just put in the neighboring room. He calls her his neighbor, she cries at night, thinking she's alone in the tears of the sickness that's starting. He goes to see her, he's barely one or two years older than she, but the sickness makes him an adult who reassures, who gives a little bit of warmth with the free hand that's left "you'll see it's not that hard, and everybody is nice around here."

He still believes in life that goes forward, in his voice, in his brown eyes. He calls you to tell you so, gives you courage. He still wants to look good, chooses his boxers and his T-shirts according to his visitors, is amazed at the coats, gloves, asks if it's cold outside, worries, asks his aunt Maya to go home "it's late, you live far away." He doesn't know that he has the grace of an angel. An angel who was asked to do homework, exercises during which Mamita cheats like she used to do when they played dominos to let him win, easy exercises because he loves the "good job" in the margin - the "GJ" like he used to say, with this voice that goes up to the summit of the achieved exploit. The child is so small, so soft with his happy air when he has done everything right.

He's a little man, the promise of a future, he has a friend, Bertille, whom he talks about, his heart full of hope, he has nothing to hide, his arms in the shape of a cross, offered.

It's what he tells the nurses as they are busy trying to put back his catheter without anesthesia: "no really this time you have to hurry up, my girlfriend is waiting for me at home, I can't disappoint her." He waits, playing, he doesn't stop playing, cards, checkers, "big pile of shit," and it's the name that cracked him up, on the game boy on which a friend tried to win him lives. He organizes soccer championships, a world cup on the screen, writes the scores, the players, and works for whole days. He doesn't like what's serious: the medical cares, take his fever, be examined "you see it's not necessary, many have done it before," he applies himself to the games, tries to finish them, listens to the advice from his guests, teaches the nurse to play checkers, card games, while learning to live in a bubble, in a sterile room: "be very careful, Mamita, if you drop a card, it's over, there will be one missing in the deck."

On my computer in memory of your messages, hundreds of messages, your name and mine repeated hundreds of times. Sometimes the emails are several pages long. Like a transfusion of words. You tell me about things that you never had time to live: the hurricane of the sickness, the emergencies you had to face without thinking, without having time to take a step back, since the next obstacle was already there and you already had to plan, cope with a new treatment, the sequence of the sickness, the successive episodes.

You tell me that it's good that I'm here in the morning, with my words when you turn your computer on, your eyes still blind. You give thanks. You tell me that you're going to help me write the book. That it's my words that made you want to come out of your isolation.

You correct some dates, narrate some moments, you say it's important, it's your story, you don't want me to dress it up, like in the theater when the actors' costumes help understanding the play, you only want the truth, naked, free of all adornments, his story as if he had to recite it in front of Osiris Tribunal for the weighing of the soul and that his heart on the scale was lighter than Maat's feather.

I follow you looking for clues, rereading your emails. I send you pages that you edit, modify. I take back my painting colors, add details, and start again.

This letter that I write with your words added to mine, I don't know what's what anymore. Only this sentence, as a backdrop, that repeats itself over and over again: I'm not here, I'm here and I would have loved so much to be here, and above it, your words that answer me, calm me down, bring me comfort, guide my hand, change a detail, complete it. You add episodes I don't know anything about and that you forgot to tell me about, insist on exceptional moments, instants of happiness, a simple breakfast shared with your two children on a Sunday morning, moments where the suffering was absent, just for a few minutes, a few hours, just the time to be conscious about happiness, to feel it flow in your souls, not only thanks to the respite given by the sickness, but for the happiness that you felt for being together. You would like me to write about it, this tenderness given for eternity not only about the bad, the pain, but also the love, yours when you came, my eternal friends, and all the people suffering should be surrounded as much, but also Sebastien's, little child, little love so generous, so fair, when he would say, "I feel better

about myself because I feel better with others."
You talk about the inspiration of the plan you had developed to make him dream, to forget the present, to give him the will to live, to draw on because it is beautiful, life is so beautiful. You relearn to live, to have activities that don't need to be canceled since everything is possible in the present, since life is an immense field, huge.

I understand the nights spent preparing with details the holidays, the escapes from the hospital taking into consideration all the various parameters, complex, tied to the treatment, to the sickness, to the child's fragility. Useless nights, from now on, even if you succeeded, deployed remarkable organization skills doubled with an energy eternally renewed by his love, yours, multiplied to the infinite.

It wasn't always easy, at first, the first weeks, every time that one of your plans failed, you sank with him, exhausted, desperate, disappointed. Quickly, you learned how to renounce, how to propose another future, another place, another date, other marvels to draw, discuss, evaluate, measure. You were for him the breath of life, you gave him a purpose, helped him accept another tomorrow, a happiness maybe, unpredictable, surprising. I try to follow you, to be faithful to you, I know the beginning and the end of the story, between the two of you, the time of the sickness as I was far away, the time of the sadness, impossible to open, that you're avoiding, that I perceive through some of your chosen words, certain adjectives that keep coming back, some pauses, some silences.

For you, I take notes, I reread paragraphs already written, take out a precision, modify, wait. I stay at the surface; I have the feeling that I have big clumsy fingers, that I go around the story without really getting it.

One night, I try to understand, to reread the emails we exchanged during the sickness, to go back before the fall, and I hurt myself: on the screen are Sebastien's words, Pierre's spelling mistakes, some fish lists for the future fishing parties at the other end of the world, promises of getting back together, your wishes for the new year that didn't come true, some big sloppy kisses signed Babar Bastien. I renounce, cry a whole evening in front of the screen because of the nickname.

One day the message I was waiting for, without knowing it, arrives.
Terrible.

A letter that nobody will ever receive from the post office. Words that can only be pronounced very quickly with your fingers on a computer, like a confession, and that you send without editing them.

I wake up one morning, I turn on my computer and, with the sunrise, the whole house bathing the morning sun, the children fighting to eat breakfast, I read it, Sebastien's last day, told with sentences, a text with a beginning and an end.

Nobody stopped you on your way, nobody saw your tears, I don't know why I imagine tears while your hands are running on the desktop, nobody took you in their arms to cease the words, even for only a minute, just time for you to comprehend the situation, the time of a shower, of a meal. No, you write to me a whole weekend, seated on your bed, the computer on your lap. Across from you, no faces, no one looking, no reaction. No glass in your hands, no coffee cup, no silence to drink a sip, no fire in the fireplace, no questions. Just you facing the screen.

You explain to me like a countdown that Saturday and that Sunday of the End. His last moments.

You had breakfast with your older son on the morning of the last Sunday in the kitchen, when you still didn't know that the minutes of the hospital were counted. This escapade you had planned with the "big one," somewhere in France, to take care a little bit of him. I notice the two words "little bit," I see there, this mother's guilt that drove you all the time to push back the limits of what was possible to do in a day, in a week and that every night, before you went to bed, made you sigh as you were writing to me because it made you accomplish more, mainly more. You wanted to listen to him, the big brother, share with him those battles, that you were fighting against the sickness, that he was fighting with you since he was encouraging him by paying attention in class, a good student, autonomous when you left him at home in the evenings.

I didn't write much about Guillaume, not that his pain is lesser, less worthy of being told but because it's another story. The story of a brother, of love and passion, of shared or revealed secrets, of compared strength, of gifts, exchanged, a constant fight to be noticed, speak, raise their voices, have the last word in the car or at the table, tell each other jokes, whisper silly things, say "it's not me, it's him," play for hours begging for a few more minutes before going to bed, laugh looking at each other in the eyes, fight in the morning because of the surprise in the cereal box, at night for the TV program: NBC, no CBS,NBC, no CBS, click on the remote while the other one is changing the channel directly on the TV set, NBC, CBS,NBC,CBS, no, yes, no, yes . . .

And it's not what I wrote about.

So, you were with your older son and you were about to leave, leaving the little one, just for a few hours, you had warned him, you would go see him on Saturday morning and right after you'd come back on Sunday night. Between the two, he wouldn't be alone, you had everything planned, his father, your family, hour by hour, timed visits, relieving troops assured, from the time he woke up to the time he went to bed.

You repeat it, you had to go, you had organized a few minutes of freedom exactly one year after the beginning of the sickness. Maybe to recoup some strength, believe in new battles, not despair, get ready for a war whose ending you wanted to believe was uncertain, in the long term, very long term, a year, maybe two . . .

When the doctors were talking about a few days, this time.

22nd of September 2001 message

Re: That day

I want to say more and more, I want to talk, not to forget. So that you know? That day, the 11th of March, but also the previous day is like we had slowly drifted towards his departure . . . Impression of a countdown. The hospital visits were always organized so that he would never be alone, so that he would have someone with him every day, from the moment he woke up to the time he went to sleep.

On that day, I had to go on a weekend to Poitiers to visit the "Futuroscope" with Guillaume. Take care of him a little. But he had a sore throat, and we canceled. On Saturday morning, I went to see Sebastien, but I stayed with the next visit: I didn't go home to take care of Guillaume; I stayed there, with him. As if it were my place. An obvious fact. No stress, no fear, just the necessity to be there, even if I didn't like that Guillaume was alone for such a long period of time, a touch of guilt but . . .

So I stayed the whole time my brother and one of his daughters were there, when they went for a walk before coming back for a little while. My mother arrived . . . I still didn't leave.

Sebastien was not talking. He was nothing else but physical pain; you couldn't touch the smallest part of his body.

When I finally decided to leave him at the end of the day, I asked the nurses to relieve him even more. What they were giving him was not enough. They were going to give him morphine and I left. He spent his last evening with Yasmine. I still haven't been able to talk about these moments with her. I just know that on that morning, he was totally absent. I called him on the phone before going to visit him. He couldn't reach for the phone, he told my aunt Maya, who was there with him, that he was not in pain anymore, that he was on a cloud, that he was gliding. He was well, calm, in peace.

That day, I hadn't organized the day's visits, I hadn't said who was going to come after me and who was going to be there in the evening. Or maybe, it's just an impression since my sister and a friend were there. On that day, what is certain is that I didn't have anything planned but to be at the hospital, the whole day, available, for him, the three of us together for as long as possible.

We had a nice breakfast with Guillaume, and we left. When I arrived, the nurses told me that his bed hadn't been made for two days since he wasn't getting up anymore. I had a roasted chicken and some gravy that the three of us were going to eat, his dream. I carried it, and left it on a chair, not to crowd the bed, I took a pan of hot water and I washed his feet with a soap made of coconut . . . I let his feet soak in the hot water a little. Pleasure.

There were the three of us, him lying on his bed without suffering, without any desire to eat, but he said that he was going to eat later. Guillaume was playing with his game boy to win him lives.

And his blood pressure dropped, he started having a hard time breathing, we asked Guillaume to leave the room.

He told me that he was going to die with his own words, with children words I didn't understand, he said: "it's the finale," and silly me, I answered him that in a finale there was a winner. He asks me to open the blinds, more, more, he wanted to see the sky and be in the light. He wasn't looking at me, I told you. He was thirsty and I put a wet compress on his lips so that he didn't make any effort, but that a few drops of water would wet his throat.

He was hot. It was complicated to take the top part of his pajamas off with all the tubes, the wires everywhere, heart, arms, nose, but I wanted to do it, he had sweat on his forehead, I dried them slowly, I didn't know that it was the end. He already had so many crises that had brought him to the resuscitation service that I thought it was just one more time and I thanked, mentally, the doctors not to take him to resuscitation, and give him the care in his bedroom . . .

And we called his father. His blood pressure went back up when his father arrived and told him that he needed him. His little heart started again for 2 or 3 minutes, but went back down very quickly to the level of before his father's arrival and then . . . things happened very slowly, without any revolt on his part, no panic on mine.

I don't think that I believed it; I hope that I gave him enough authorization to leave.

I have one regret, only one. At one point, the doctor asked to talk to us, she told us that he didn't have much time left. But she told us the same thing two weeks ago. His father asked questions, was trying to understand . . . and me I just wanted to go back to him, it wasn't interesting to me, I just wanted to accompany him, not be revolted, not deny it, not flee . . . accompany him to the end of my love, to the end of his life, to the beginning of somewhere else, something else, something different.

Here you go. The feeling that I lost two precious minutes, wanting to go back next to him instead of listening to the rational and objective conversa-

tions that didn't make any more sense. I should have gone. I didn't do it. Not a problem!!! Sebastien would have said.

When we went back into the room, it is already more blurry in my memory, I went very quickly next to him after the usual precautions: hands washed up to the elbows, mask, blouse . . . His stepmother was next to him. His father stayed in the entrance: we couldn't be more than two in his bedroom, but the right thing to do didn't exist for me anymore at that time. I went over to him and there I think that it was over very very quickly. Just the time to come back next to him, to sit on the chair, to hold his hand. He suffocated right away, he had hiccups of life or death, I don't know: I thought he was dead, gone, and suddenly his body would rise a little bit and his eyes would open. I didn't know when death happens, if these hiccups are cries for life or death.

After that I don't know anymore, I think that I cried, my head on the doctor's chest, the one who was next to me and who was comforting me.

I took all the wires off, all of them, but the perfusion, all the traces of failed life saving. And I put his pajamas back on.

After they asked me to choose some clothes, I took out some nice clothes, but I changed my mind, I decided to leave him in his favorite pajamas; the ones he loved so much and he had chosen to wear on that weekend.

They asked me to go out, his father and I left the room to announce to Guillaume that it was over. My sister arrived and I comforted her, we had coffee, stunned, in an office prepared for us by the medical team.

I was asked to go back.

It was in shock: the room had become cold. Nevertheless it was the same room, I recognized the walls, the bed, but this room in which we had fought so hard for life a few minutes earlier, this room full of agitation and the sounds of machines had become empty. Only the silence, the stiff body, inert, with all the members at the right place, with a trace of interrupted movement, in order, with this sheet stretched from the toes, aligned, raised, up to the beginning of the shoulders.

For a very long time I thought that it was inhumane to let the parents see that. And then, a short time later, I told myself that it was an inevitable step, a real way to make me realize that his body was not alive anymore.

I never expect to see him come out of his school again. I never expect to see his look again.

I put on his little body the feather Laurent had brought

him, the one he used to chase the sickness away from his body, with a movement that Laurent must have shown him.

OK, I'm going to stop.
Big kisses, all naked inside, without any protection.
Love the ones who love you and whom you love.
See you later to share a life maybe more recent.
Nat.

I don't answer you right away. I can't touch any of your words, disturb their order, and detach them. I cry at the unspeakable that you managed to tell me, I cry at the heartfelt trust that you give me, all the way in my womb.

Mothers.

I thank you, like there's nothing left to say.

You're the one who writes:

That last day of Seb, I have lived it night and day, a hundred times, for months.
To not forget.
To try to see what I maybe hadn't seen before.
And one day when I wrote to you, my memory was freed . . .
He was not in the forefront anymore, I could make him come back when I wanted, he didn't need to

come back into my memory in spite of me, without me calling him.

You continue to write to me. I realize that the letters you write to me are the ones you would write if you had to die.

You read dozens of books on death, sickness, and books about life, about death. I picture you in Paris, under the covers, for entire weekends, in October. I try to remember: October, the month of October, the October rain. I try to find objective reasons to this sudden imprisonment.

You send me book extracts that you read and you write to me with a flowing writing, immediate, that comes directly from your soul. You keep the computer open on the top of your thighs, you don't leave your bed, with only the wet light of Paris' roofs. Wet, I don't know, the simple light, gray, white, blue, the light, that you barely see since you're sitting on a mattress right on the carpet. It's not that you're poor, you're not, but you never bought a bed. Sleeping at your place has always been a reason to joke around about sleeping on the floor. But I have liked your bed ever since the night I arrived and we all carried our mattresses on the carpet of your room.

For me it's morning, for you it's already the evening,

we are like Queen Victoria ruling an empire that never sleeps: between us two, the day, the night, good morning, good night, the day goes on, life goes on, death tamed, the intimate life.

You want to start anew, to clean everything, to see yourself live, see yourself die. You want to enter all the worlds, push all the doors, build playrooms for the youth, the adolescents, the old, the elders in retirement homes, day nurseries, put all of them together.

You can't bear loneliness anymore. You can't accept lonely children in hospitals anymore, lonely men and women because they're afraid, of sickness, of pain, of death, of talking. You would like hospitals to be humane. Schools and companies too.

You would like people to talk to each other, to love each other, to help each other live and die.

You would like to thank, and you don't know how, everyone who has helped you, helped Sebastien, so they know that they have been precious. You would like them to go back again and again in the sick children's room, in the forgotten children's room, the ones nobody wants to see, in the tall walls' shadow, in the labyrinth of services, of floors, and halls. Above all, you want them to start coming again, to invite themselves in children's eyes, to tear apart their boredom, to give them words for food.

You show me a picture, you say "David Douillet," Sebastien looks thrilled, stunned to be suddenly back in the world, to be more lucky than his friends, to be able to talk, for once, about something else than the disease.

You talk about those who took him to a soccer game at the "Stade de France" in the official grandstand, suddenly, the joy, Versailles, all the colors of life lit in his eyes. All the trust of a child who was a captain again, dressed in his team's jersey, for the game of his life, on his bed.

You write the draft of a letter to thank them all. A letter gift. You list the people you have to send it to. You would like it to be beautiful, even the stamps that you have chosen, "thank-you" stamps and charity stamps, two small Marian stamps and a rectangular stamp to form a square. You write a hundred and eleven messages on a piece of paper made of hope, then you collapse, exhausted, because there's nothing left to do when you have said thank you. A few people answer you.

A little while before Christmas, I come back. It's so simple, a day on a plane, 12 hours on the way in, 12 hours on the way out to stay 4 days with you. Finish the book, be by your side before the certainty of Sebastien's absence in front of the illuminated Christmas tree.

You ask me if I have questions. I'm so happy to be with you that I don't have any questions, seeing you again, no questions for the wind that blows in the streets of Paris as we are walking hand in hand, avoiding the craziness of the department stores and the Christmas decorations, no questions to ask the silence when I can finally hold you in my arms, communicate differently from my computer's keypad and the endless emails. We talk late into the night, in a café, at the restaurant, sitting on the bed, the couch. I have a thousand questions to ask you, but I don't ask one. I would like to understand without you having to explain, relieve your memory without asking you to talk. You understand it, you help me as much as you can, you entrust me with a plastic bag in which you put away the letters of testimony of parents or friend answering your letter. All the messages are neatly folded, saved in their envelopes. Gathered. Like antidotes on a desperate day.

I give these manuscripts the same care I used to

give my studies, while I was writing my thesis, and reading philosophy books. I practice paleography, I decipher handwritings, letters, for some only a few sentences jotted down randomly on paper, in pencil, in a hurry. Pain that we try to contain. For others, words carefully copied after a first draft, in which the tears of their voices were erased. Many don't say anything, only conventional words, pre-owned words. The words that we say ordinarily without giving out too much of ourselves. And here and there, some islands of the heart. The doctor from the beginning, the one who had shared with him a jar of pickles in the hospital parking lot after weeks of isolation, who talks about therapeutic failure with the sadness of a woman, not of a doctor, a note from a social worker who signs "his hospital auntie." Your sister Pitou and her friend Marc who, without talking to each other, both talk about the joy to carry Sebastien, adorable weight. Seb as a child, his face lost in a big blue hat with white fur who holds your sister with his little arms as she is carrying him, in the mountains, proud to be his favorite, Marc who offers the nest of his shoulders for Seb's last stroll in the forest, without knowing that the child is scared to fall and gives him his complete trust and acceptance. Catherine, your older sister who writes a letter to express her

pain, her difficulty to share it. But who does it any-
way, evoking this magical place that is Tharon,
where Seb as a child, was participating to the life
of this big family that you are. Fragile links we remember, with emotion. Promise of a future. Baby
with diapers and a bottle, first words, astonishment
in the kitchen of the grown ups. Always the same
story of men, from childbirth to death, never with
the same episodes nor the same loves. Finally your
brother Thierry who, the last one, the most timid,
brings you a poem about tenderness, suffering, and
the serenity of the last pictures.

The eternity of the love narrated with soft words
whose details touch my soul. Your mother's words
that I carefully caress with an infinite respect. They
only speak of the perpetual love for the child. The
child adult, you, her daughter, the child-child,
Sebastien.

A few hours before my departure, you sit on my
bed, the breakfast just finished, and you tell me
that you're going to correct my story, try to find for
me a path on the ocean of your sadness, tell me
what I don't know, walk on water.

You get out your calendars, the calendar of this
year ending and the other, the year of the sickness

agenda, you open them in the palm of your hands, flat, in front of you and you start to talk. I quickly take a few sheets of paper and, without a word, I take notes, I obey your voice, I go over to your side. Outside, it's Sunday, I write, I fill in dozens of pages, as if you were dictating them.

Facing me, on the bedroom's wall, in a frame, a black and yellow poster: a Tuareg is pouring tea in a tiny cup. I see his hand, too big, beyond measure, laying on the coffee maker like fingers on a bow and the thread of brown liquid fall into the tiny cup. I hear the sound of the water, it's the same as your voice, a tiny thread, but precise, that falls exactly in the palm of my hand, exactly between the thumb and the forefinger when I hold the pen. The tea is poured in a slow serenity, a tranquil trajectory. I become an instrument, a scribe, a chronicler, I adapt to your voice. I listen, hypnotized, at the same time, by your vivid wound, being narrated, the memory being emptied and the friendship you demonstrate towards me, you're able to pour it like a brown tea on white pages.

Sometimes, when your voice stops, I pretend I'm writing, so that you continue, that the miracle happens, your words continue to flow, get closer to me. Far from everything. Far from that Sunday when we won't live. Because we're somewhere else in a time machine, a time that goes by, page after page in the calendar, in a present where words are witnesses, hospital names, missed appointments, meetings that never happened, a present interrupted by crisis, warnings, where each second of life was precious. You lean over the yellow pages of your diary, like you did over Seb's bed in the light of your love.

You take your time. You go over pages where you haven't said everything. You explain. It's difficult to explain love at the edge of the abyss.

I'm quiet. I ask very few questions. I'm afraid that you're about to lose it, that it will stop, that you will not finish your sentences. You're not looking at me; you're looking at him, somewhere else. Sometimes, I force you to jump. I tell you that I know, that I will find it again. Sometimes, I'm the one who gives precision.

It's late; the daylight is starting to fade. You're quiet. You just stumbled on Sebastien's last day as if it were the last limit.

It's over. You're empty. You stay a long time in my arms, without moving, in the present. I smile at you. You haven't said everything, you will never be finished telling.

But for the rest, you just have to live.

To go on, in pain and in happiness, day by day.

Together we look at Sebastien's tape, with a warm thought for the young man who brought it in a hurry the day before the funeral. We had watched it then, because, before the ceremony, you wanted to make sure that Seb hadn't left you a secret message in it. You wanted to be as close as possible to him, catch one of his looks and tell him that he was a smart cookie one last time.

I realize that I know his words almost by heart and they're almost the same as yours. I'm thinking that he's succeeding: you're not separated anymore, he doesn't send any messages, he's your heart being reconciled, tied in you, caressed, in you, the shadow and the light more complete, in you the visible and invisible connected, life found again. I think that you're succeeding, with a heart ready to give, to cure, a live heart, bigger, an infinitely big heart that will grow even more with the endless desire to love.

On the plane, I open the package you gave me. It's a perfume bottle, yours. A silent presence. I put a little bit on. Now and then, I close my eyes, I smell the back of my hand, and I smell you.

On the card, you wrote: an extract from Sebastien's interview: "If you had a message to give the sick children in the hospitals or the ones who are starting their treatment, what would you say to them?"

It would be to fight, and at the end, the result, it will be great, and they will be free.

I smile, my eyes wet. It must be the jetlag. "You're not very comforted," Seb whispers in my ears, making fun of me.

GREEN INTEGER
Pataphysics and Pedantry

Douglas Messerli, *Publisher*

Essays, Manifestos, Statements, Speeches, Maxims,
Epistles, Diaristic Notes, Narratives, Natural Histories,
Poems, Plays, Performances, Ramblings, Revelations
and all such ephemera as may appear necessary
to bring society into a slight tremolo of confusion
and fright at least.

*

GREEN INTEGER TITLES